TY

VENTRIC
- Precordial th...
- Defibrillate 2(
- Defibrillate 3(
- Defibrillate 36
- ET & IV acce...

MW01045551

- Epinephrine 1 ... , ... q ... min
- Defibrillate 360¹J
- Consider alternate Epi dosing †
- Administer class IIa drugs
- Defibrillate 360 J 30-60 sec after each med (drug-shock pattern)
- Consider Bicarbonate 1 meq/kg †

CLASS IIA DRUGS†
- Lidocaine 1-1.5 mg/kg² IVP may repeat 1.5 mg/kg in 3-5 min up to 3 mg/kg loading dose
- Bretylium 5 mg/kg, then repeat 10 mg/kg in 5 min²
- $MgSO_4$ 1-2 g over 1-2 min³
- Procainamide 30 mg/min up to 17 mg/kg in refractory VF²

¹Defibrillate within 30-60 sec after med; may give multiple sequenced shocks here, especially when meds are delayed.
²Post resuscitation drip rates: Lidocaine 2-4 mg/min, Bretylium 1-2 mg/min, Procainamide 1-4 mg/min.
³Use in torsades de pointes, suspected low Mg levels, or severe refractory Ventricular Fibrillation (VF)

VENTRICULAR ECTOPY
- O_2, IV access
- Rule out treatable causes:
  - Acidosis   • Alkalosis
  - Hypoxemia   • Digoxin toxicity
  - Bradycardia
  - Other drug toxicities
  - Electrolyte imbalance
- Lidocaine 1 mg/kg IVP, Repeat at 0.5 mg/kg q 3-5 min
- Procainamide 20-30 mg/min IV

- Acidosis (see bicarbonate note)
- Tension pneumothorax (needle decompression)
- Cardiac tamponade (pericardiocentesis)
- Hypoxemia (ventilation)
- Hypovolemia (volume infusion)
- Hypothermia (see algorithm)
- Drug overdose (specific therapy)
- Hyperkalemia ($NaHCO_3^-$, $CaCl_2$)
- Massive Acute Myocardial Infarction
- If cause is not identified, then,
  - Epinephrine 1 mg q IVP 3-5 min AND/OR
  - Atropine 1mg IVP q 3-5 min (for absolute or relative bradycardia)

DDX of PEA:
- EMD   • Pseudo-EMD
- Bradyasystolic rhythms
- Idioventricular rhythms
- Ventricular escape rhythms
- Post-defib idioventricular rhythms

ASYSTOLE
- ET & IV access ASAP
- Confirm in more than one lead
- Consider causes:
  - Preexisting acidosis • Hypoxia
  - Hypokalemia   • Hyperkalemia
  - Drug overdose   • Hypothermia
- Consider Transcutaneous pacing [1 b] (must be initiated early)
- Epinephrine 1mg IVP q 3-5 min
- Atropine 1mg IVP q 3-5 min
- Physician may consider termination of efforts after intubation, initial meds, & no reversible causes are found. Also, consider arrest time.

---

†See page 4 for more information on specific drug administration & other information

BRADYCARDIA

- O₂, IV access
- Assess vital signs & rhythm[1]

SERIOUS SIGNS OR SYMPTOMS[2] PRESENT:

- Atropine[3] 0.5-1 mg q 3-5 min [I & IIa]
- Transcutaneous pacer [I]†
- Dopamine 5-20 mcg/kg/min [IIb] †
- Epinephrine 2-10 mcg/min [IIb]
- Isoproterenol[4]

ASYMPTOMATIC 2° TYPE II OR 3° AV HEART BLOCK[5]:

- Transvenous pacer †
  (may use TCP as bridge device)

ASYMPTOMATIC NOT 2° Type II or 3°

- Observe

[1] Is rhythm sinus, AV block, &/or wide complex?
[2] Signs: shock, hypotension, pulmonary congestion, CHF, acute MI.
Symptoms: chest pain, SOB, decreased LOC. Do not delay pacing while waiting for drugs!
[3] Total dose is 0.04mg/kg. Consider shorter dosing in severe conditions. Use with caution in Type II 2° & new 3° AV nodal blocks with wide QRS - may worsen block; pacing is always appropriate. Transplanted hearts will not respond to atropine - must use pacer &/or epi. Atropine may worsen ischemia or induce VT&/or VF if acute MI is present.
[4] Use with extreme caution - at low doses is IIb, at higher doses is III.
[5] Never use lidocaine in 3° AV block with ventricular escape beats.

ACUTE MI

- INITIAL ASSESSMENT
  Immediate: • Vital signs with auto BP
  - O₂% saturation, IV, 12-lead
  - Brief, targeted Hx & physical
  - Eligibility for thrombolytics
  Soon: • CXR, blood work, consult PRN
- TREATMENT OPTIONS
  - O₂ AT 4 L/min   • PTCA
  - Nitroglycerin SL (if SBP >90)
  - Morphine IV†   • Aspirin PO
  - Thrombolytics   • Nitroglycerin IV†
  - β-blockers IV†   • Heparin IV
  - Lidocaine routine use is *not* recommended

HYPOTENSION, SHOCK & ACUTE PULMONARY EDEMA

- O₂, IV access
- Assess vital signs, history & patient

RATE PROBLEM:

- Go to appropriate algorithm

VOLUME PROBLEM:

- Administer fluids, blood as needed, cause-specific interventions, & finally consider vasopressors as BP dictates.
- SBP <70 mmHg & signs of shock
  Consider Norepinephrine 0.5 mcg/min†
  or Dopamine 5-20mcg/kg/min† (wean norepinephrine & replace with dopamine as BP improves)
- SBP 70-100mmHg & signs of shock
  Dopamine 2.5-20 mcg/kg/min†
  (add norepinephrine if dopamine >20)
- SBP >100 mmHg & normal DBP
  Dobutamine 2-20 mcg/kg/min†
- DBP >110 mmHg
  Start Nitroglycerin 10-20 mcg/min IV†
  (may titrate to effect) OR
  Nitroprusside at 0.1-5 mcg/kg/min †

ACUTE PULMONARY EDEMA:

- First line actions:
  - Furosemide IV 0.5-1 mg/kg
  - Morphine IV 1-3 mg †
  - Nitroglycerin SL
  - O₂ / intubate PRN
- Second line actions:
  - Nitroglycerin IV (if SBP>100)†
  - Nitroprusside IV (if SBP>100)†
  - Dopamine (if SBP<100)†
  - Dobutamine (if SBP>100)†
  - PEEP or CPAP
- Third line actions:
  - Amrinone 0.75 mg/kg/min †
  - Aminophylline 5 mg/kg
    (if wheezing)
  - Thrombolytic therapy (if no shock)
  - Digoxin (if A. fib or SVT)†
  - Angioplasty
  - IABP
  - Open Heart Surgery

---

†See page 4 for more information on specific drug administration & other information

TACHYCARDIA
- O_2, IV access
- Assess vital signs
- Treat pulseless VT as VF

•**If unstable with serious signs, symptoms[1] → proceed with cardioversion.**
•**If stable → Attempt to identify rhythm further & proceed with appropriate algorithm listed below.**

Paroxysmal Supraventricular Tachycardia (PSVT)
- Vagal maneuvers[2]
- Adenosine 6 mg IVP over 1-3 sec
- Adenosine 12 mg IVP over 1-3 sec (may repeat in 1-2 min)
- PSVT complex width? Narrow or Wide

Narrow PSVT complex width
- If *unstable*- synchronized cardioversion (see below)
- If *stable*, proceed with the following:
- Verapamil 2.5-5mg IVP
- Verapamil 5-10 mg IVP 15-30min after first dose †
- Consider digoxin,β-blockers,diltiazem
- Synchronized cardioversion(see below)

Wide PSVT complex width
- Lidocaine 1-1.5 mg/kg IVP
- Procainamide 20-30 mg/min
- Synchronized cardioversion (see below)

Atrial fibrillation or flutter
- Consider use of: †

•diltiazem	•β-blockers
•verapamil	•digoxin
•procainamide	•quinidine
•anticoagulants	

Wide Complex Tachycardia of Uncertain Type
- Lidocaine 1-1.5mg/kg IVP then 0.5-0.75mg/kg IVP q5-10 min up to 3mg/kg
- Adenosine 6mg IVP over 1-3 sec
- Adenosine 12mg IVP over 1-3 sec (may repeat in 1-2 min)
- Procainamide 20-30 mg/min
- Bretylium 5-10 mg/kg
- Synchronized cardioversion
- Start drip with last used antiarrhythmic.

Ventricular Tachycardia (VT)
- Lidocaine 1-1.5mg/kg IVP, then 0.5-0.75mg/kg IVP q5-10min. Max 3 mg/kg
- Procainamide 20-30 mg/min
- Bretylium 5-10 mg/kg
- Synchronized cardioversion
- Start drip with last used antiarrhythmic

Torsades de pointes
- Overdrive pacing †-treatment of choice
- $MgSO_4$ 1-2g IV over 1-2 min.
- Isoproterenol 2-10 mcg/min may overdrive the ventricular rate.

Cardioversion
- If ventricular rate >150 bpm prepare for immediate cardioversion, may give brief trial of meds based on rhythm. Cardioversion is generally not needed for rates <150 bpm.
- ✓O_2 sat, IV, prepare to intubate
- Sedate when possible[3]
- Synchronized cardioversion[4]

VT [5]	•100J then,
PSVT [6]	•200J then,
Atrial fibrillation	•300J then,
Atrial flutter [6]	•360J

[1]*Signs*: shock, hypotension, pulmonary congestion, CHF, acute MI *Symptoms*: chest pain, shortness of breath, Decreased LOC
[2]Vagal maneuvers consist of carotid massage (unless cerebrovascular disease or carotid bruit present), breath holding, coughing, NG tube placement, gag reflex stimulation, eyeball pressure, squatting, Mast trousers, Trendelenburg's position, Valsalva, "diving reflex" (unless ischemic heart disease),circumferential sweep of the anus.
[3]Possible sedatives: diazepam, midazolam, barbiturates, etomidate, ketamine, methohexital. Possible analgesia: fentanyl, morphine, meperidine
[4]If synchronization is delayed & clinical situation is critical, go immediately to un-synchronized
[5]Treat polymorphic VT like VF.
[6]PSVT & atrial flutter often respond to 50J.

CLASSIFICATION OF THERAPEUTIC OPTIONS

Class I: usually indicated, always acceptable, & considered useful & effective. (Definitely helpful)

Class II: acceptable, of uncertain efficacy, & may be controversial.

Class IIa: the weight of evidence is in favor of its usefulness & efficacy. (Acceptable, probably helpful)

Class IIb: not well established by evidence, yet may be helpful & is probably not harmful. (Acceptable, possibly helpful)

Class III: is inappropriate, is without scientific supporting data, & may be harmful. (Not indicated, may be harmful)

ACLS MEDICATIONS

adenosine [Adenocard]: (6 mg/2 ml) IV initial dose 6 mg over 1-2 sec, then 12 mg within 1-2 min if needed, 12 mg may be repeated once if needed; follow the rapid IV bolus by 20cc saline flush; theophylline is antagonistic. Adenosine depresses AV & SA node activity only. Half-life is <5 sec.

amrinone [Inocor]: Initial bolus 0.75 mcg/kg IV over 2-3 min, followed by 5-15 mcg/kg/min infusion.

atropine: 0.5-1.0 mg IVP q 3-5 min. Maximum dose is 0.03-0.04 mg/kg which produces complete vagal block.

β-Blockers: atenolol - 5-10 mg IV over 5 min. metoprolol - 5-10 mg slow IVP q 5 min to a total of 15 mg. Then 50 mg PO BID for at least 24 hrs, then increase to 100 mg BID. propranolol - 0.1 mg/kg in 3 divided doses, give slow IVP at 2-3 min intervals. Then 180-320 mg/day PO in divided doses.

bretylium: Load with 5-10 mg/kg SIVP, maintain at 2-4 mg/min IV; MAX 35 mg/kg. In persistent VT, dilute 5-10 mg/kg in 50cc D$_5$W and inject IV over 8-10 min.

calcium: Class IIa with hyperkalemia, Ca^{2+}- channel blocker toxicity, hypocalcemia; otherwise it is Class III. When necessary use 2-4 mg/kg of 10% CaCl$_2$ q 10 min as needed or 5-8 ml of calcium gluconate

diltiazem: [Cardizem Injectable] 20 mg (0.25 mg/kg) over 2 min, then 25 mg (0.35 mg/kg) if needed in 15 min, then 5-15 mg/hr IV infusion for up to 24h can be used to control Atrial Fibrillation rate.

dobutamine: Usual dose is 2-20 mcg/kg/min. (1000mg in 250cc D$_5$W or NS). Heart rate increases, especially at higher doses - this may exacerbate myocardial ischemia.

dopamine: Add 400mg to 250ml D$_5$W (1600 mcg/ml); doses of 2-6 mcg/kg/min IV drip are predominately dopaminergic & β-agonist; doses >10 mcg/kg/min are α-agonist.

epinephrine: As vasopressor dose, 1mg in 500ml D$_5$W or NS & start with 1mcg/min continuous IV drip titrated to response. During cardiac arrest, epi may be given as a continuous infusion - add 30mg epi to 250ml D$_5$W or NS & run at 100ml/hr (comparable to the standard 1 mg dose).

Alternate Epinephrine dosing regimens: Intermediate: 2-5 mg q 3-5 min; Escalating: 1 mg, then 3 mg, then 5 mg 3min apart; High: epi 0.1 mg/kg q 3-5 min

isoproterenol: 1 mg in 500ml D$_5$W (2 mcg/ml). Low dose is 2-10 mcg/min IV drip. Titrate to heart rate & rhythm

<u>lidocaine</u>: 1-1.5 mg/kg IVP, may repeat at 0.5-1.5 mg/kg q 3-5 min, maximum dose is 3 mg/kg. Add 2 g in 250cc D5W (8 mg/ml) for IV drip.

<u>magnesium</u>: Dilute 1-2 grams in 100ml D5W & give IVP over 1-2 min in VF/VT. In patients with documented Mg deficiency, load with 1-2 g in 50-100 ml D5W give over 5-60 mins & follow with infusion of 0.5-1 g/hr up to 24h.

<u>morphine sulfate</u>: 1-3 mg IVP q 5 min. Prn analgesic of choice for acute MI, Class IIb for pulmonary edema.

<u>nitroglycerin</u>: 50 or 100 mg in 250cc D5W or NS, start at 10-20 mcg/min IV drip, increased by 5-10 mcg/min q 5-10 min. Low doses = mainly venodilation; high doses = arteriolar dilation also.

<u>nitroprusside</u>: 50-100 mg in 250cc D5W or NS (wrap solution & tubing in opaque material). IV at 0.5-10 mcg/kg/min

<u>norepinephrine</u>: Add 4 mg norepinephrine (16 mcg/ml) or 8 mg norepinephrine bitartrate (32 mcg/ml) to 250 ml D5W with or without saline; begin with 0.5-1 mcg/min IV drip & titrate.

<u>procainamide</u>: Add 1000 mg to 50cc D5W (20 mg/ml); 20-30 mg/min(1-1.5 cc/min) IV; MAX: 17 mg/kg, or 50% widening of QRS, or hypotension; 1-4 mg/min maintenance: 1000 mg in 500 ml (0.5-2 ml/min); in 250 ml (0.25-1 ml/min) Avoid use in preexisting prolonged QT interval & Torsades.

<u>sodium bicarbonate</u>: *Class I*: known preexisting hyperkalemia; *Class IIa*: preexisting HCO3 responsive acidosis; Tricyclic overdose, to alkalinize the urine in drug OD's; *Class IIb*: if intubated & long arrest interval continues, upon return of spontaneous circulation after prolonged arrest.; *Class III*: hypoxic lactic acidosis.

<u>verapamil</u>: 2.5-5 mg IVP, then 5-10 mg 15-30 min after first dose if needed. Maximum dose is 20 mg. Give only to narrow- complex PSVT or known supraventricular arrhythmias.

INDICATIONS FOR EMERGENT & STANDBY PACING
Emergent
- Hemodynamically compromised bradycardias
- Bradycardia with malignant escape rhythm
- Overdrive pacing of refractory tachycardia
- Pacing is not routinely recommended in bradyasystolic cardiac arrest - if used at all, it should be used early.

Standby
- Stable bradycardias
- Prophylactic pacing in Acute MI- Symptomatic sinus node dysfunction; Type II 2°AV nodal block; 3° AV nodal block; Newly acquired: LBBB, RBBB, alternating BBB, or bifascicular block

★★The information provided above is advisory only. This outline is not intended to take the place of complete ACLS training ★★

ACLS Notes:

ANALGESICS

ACETAMINOPHEN COMBINATIONS

Patient's age & overall clinical condition (i.e. renal and hepatic failure) should be considered when dosing narcotic containing analgesics

<u>acetaminophen supp.</u> OTC [Tylenol] (120, 325, 650 mg) PR Adult 650 mg q4-6h, >6y 325 mg q4-6h, 3-6y 120 mg q4-6h prn pain/fever

<u>acetaminophen tablets/caplets/liquid</u> OTC[Tylenol](Tab 325, 500 mg; Elx 500 mg/15ml) PO 325-1000 mg q6-8h

<u>acetaminophen Children's chewable/elixir/drops</u> OTC [Tylenol] (Tab 80, 160 mg; Elx 160 mg/5ml, 80 mg/0.8ml)
See table below for dosage

15 mg/kg/dose AGE	0-3m	4-11m	12-23m	2-3y	4-5y	6-8y	9-10y	11-12y
Drops ml q4h	0.4	0.8	1.2	1.6	2.4			
Elixir ml q4h		2.5	3.75	5	7.5	10	12.5	15
Chewable Tablets q4h				2	3	4	5	6

<u>acetylcysteine</u> [Mucomyst] *acetaminophen toxicity*: loading PO or NGT 140 mg/kg of 20% solution, then 70 mg/kg q4h x 17 doses

<u>Anexsia</u> C3 [hydrocodone/acetaminophen] (Tab 5/500, 7.5/650 mg) PO 1-2 5/500 or 1 7.5/650 mg tab q4-6h, MAX 8 & 6 tabs/24h respectively.

<u>Darvocet</u> C4 [propoxyphene/acetaminophen] (Tab N-50 50/325 mg, N-100 100/650mg) PO 1-2 N-50 or 1 N-100 tab q4h prn pain. MAX propoxyphene napsylate 600 mg/24h

<u>Esgic</u> [butalbital/acetaminophen/caffeine] (Tab 50/325/40, Plus 50/500/40 mg) PO 1 tab q4h, MAX 6 tabs/24h

<u>Fioricet</u> [butalbital/acetaminophen/caffeine] (Tab 50/325/40 mg) PO 1-2 tabs q4h, MAX 6 tabs/24h

<u>Fioricet with codeine</u> C3 [codeine/butalbital/caffeine/acetaminophen] (Tab 30/50/40/ 325 mg) PO 1-2 tabs q4h, MAX 6 tabs/24h

<u>Lorcet</u> C3 [hydrocodone 10 mg/acetaminophen 650] Tab q6h. MAX 6 tabs/24h

<u>Lortab</u> C3 [hydrocodone/acetaminophen] (Elx 2.5/120/Alcohol 7%/5ml; Tab 2.5/500, 5/500, 7.5/500 mg) PO Elx 15 ml q4h; Tab PO 1-2 2.5/500 or 5/500 tabs q4-6h. MAX 8 tabs/24h or 1 7.5/500 tab q4-6h MAX 6 tabs/24h

<u>Midrin</u> [isomethoptene/dichloralphenazone/acetaminophen] *Migraine*- PO 2 tabs then 1qh until relief, MAX 5 tabs/24h; Muscle tension- PO 1-2 q4h MAX 8 tabs/24h

<u>Norco</u> [hydrocodone/acetaminophen] (Tab 10 mg /325 mg) 1 tab q6h PRN pain. Max 6/D.

<u>Percocet</u> C2 [oxycodone/acetaminophen] (Tab 5/325 mg) PO 1 tab q6h

<u>Talacen</u> C4 [pentazocine/acetaminophen] (Tab 25/650 mg) PO 1 tab q4h, MAX 6 tabs/24h

<u>Tylenol with codeine</u> C3 [codeine/acetaminophen] (Tab [#2] 15/300, [#3] 30/300, [#4] 60/300 mg; Elx C4 12/120 mg(/5ml) adults: PO 15-60/300-1000 mg q4h, MAX 360/4000 mg/24h; Peds >3yoa: codeine 0.5 mg/kg TID/QID (3-6y 5ml, 7-12y 10ml PO TID/QID)

<u>Tylox</u> C2 [oxycodone/acetaminophen] (Tab 5/500 mg) PO 1 tab q6h

<u>Vicodin</u> C3 [hydrocodone/acetaminophen] (Tab 5/500 mg, ES 7.5/750 mg) PO 1-2 tab q4-6h,MAX 8 tabs/24h; ES 1 tab q4-6h, MAX 5 tabs/24h

<u>Wygesic</u> C4 [propoxyphene/acetaminophen] (Tab 65/650 mg) PO 1 tab q4h, MAX propoxyphene 390 mg/24h

ASPIRIN COMBINATIONS

<u>Anacin</u> OTC [ASA/caffeine] (Tab 400/32, Max 500/32 mg) PO 1-2 tabs q4h, MAX 4 gm/24h

<u>Ascriptin</u> OTC [ASA/Mg/Al hydroxide] (Tab 325/50/50 mg) PO 2-3 tabs QID, MAX 12 tabs/24h

<u>Ascriptin ES</u> OTC [ASA/Mg/Al hydroxide] (Tab 500/80/80 mg) PO 2 tabs TID/QID, MAX 8 tabs/24h

<u>Damason-P</u> C3 [hydrocodone/ASA] (Tab 5/500 mg) PO 1-2 tabs q4-6h, MAX 8 tabs/24h

<u>Darvon Compound-65</u> C4 [propoxyphene/ASA/caffeine] (Tab 65/389/32.4 mg) PO 1 tab q4h, MAX propoxyphene 390 mg/24h

<u>Equagesic</u> C4 [ASA/meprobamate] (Tab 325/200 mg) PO 1-2 tabs TID/QID

<u>Fiorinal</u> C3 [butalbital/caffeine/ASA] (Tab & Caps 50/40/325 mg) PO 1-2 tabs q4h, MAX 6 tabs/24h

<u>Fiorinal with codeine</u> C3 [codeine/butalbital/caffeine/ASA] (Tab 30/50/40/325 mg) PO 1-2 tabs q4h, MAX 6 tabs/24h

<u>Lortab ASA</u> C3 [hydrocodone/ASA] (Tab 5/500 mg) PO 1-2 tabs q4-6h, MAX 8 tabs/24h

<u>Norgesic</u> [orphenadrine/ASA/caffeine] (Tab 25/385/30 mg) PO 1-2 tabs TID/QID

<u>Norgesic Forte</u> [orphenadrine/ASA/caffeine] (Tab 50/770/60 mg) PO 0.5-1 tab TID/QID

<u>Percodan</u> C2 [oxycodone/ASA] (Tab 4.5/325 mg) PO 1 tab q6h

<u>Robaxisal</u> [methocarbamol/ASA] (Tab 400/325 mg) PO 2 tabs QID

<u>SOMA Compound</u> [carisoprodol/ASA] (Tab 200/325 mg) PO 1-2 tabs QID (>12yoa)

<u>SOMA Compound with Codeine</u> C3 [carisoprodol/ASA/codeine] (Tab 200/325/16 mg) PO 1-2 tabs QID (>12yoa)

<u>Talwin Compound</u> C4 [pentazocine/ASA] (Tab 12.5/325 mg) PO 2 tabs TID/QID (>12yoa only)

MUSCLE RELAXANTS

baclofen [Lioresal] (Tab 10, 20 mg; Amps 10 mg/5ml,10 mg/20ml) PO 5 mg TID, titrate up by 5 mg q3 D to effect
carisoprodol [Soma] (Tab 350 mg) PO 350 mg TID and at HS
chlorzoxazone [Parafon Forte DSC] (Tab 500 mg) PO 500-750 mg TID/QID
cyclobenzaprine [Flexeril] (Tab 10 mg) PO 10 mg TID, MAX 60 mg/24h
dantrolene [Dantrium] (Tab 25, 50,100 mg) PO 25 QD, titrate up to 100 mg QID, MAX 400 mg/24h
diazepam *C4* [Valium] (Tab 2, 5, 10 mg) PO 2-10 mg TID/QID
flavoxate [Urispas] (Tab 100 mg) PO 100-200 mg TID/QID, (>12yoa)
metaxalone [Skelaxin] (Tab 400 mg) *>12yoa use* 800 mg 3-4 times daily
methocarbamol [Robaxin] (Tab 500, 750 mg) PO 1-1.5g QID; IV 1-3g <3ml/m, IM ≤500mg in each gluteal region
orphenadrine [Norflex] (Tab 100 mg) IV/IM 60 mg BID, PO 100 mg BID
tizanidine [Zanaflex] (Tab 4 mg) 4-8 mg q6-8h; Start - 4 mg and titrate to effect (Max 3 doses or 36 mg /24h)

NARCOTIC EQUIVALENCE CHART

Generic	Trade	Schedule[a]	Duration[b]	t½ hrs	PO	IM/IV[c]
buprenorphine	Buprenex	V	4-6h	6-12	N/A	0.3mg
butorphanol	Stadol	N/A	3-4h	2.5-3.5	N/A	2 mg
codeine		III	4-6h	3-4	200 mg	120 mg
fentanyl	Sublimaze	II	1-2h	3-4	N/A	0.1mg
hydromorphone	Dilaudid	II	4-5h	2-3	7.5 mg	1.5 mg
levorphanol	Levo-Dromoran	II	6-8h	12-16	2 mg	4 mg
meperidine	Demerol	II	2-4h	3-4	300 mg	75 mg
methadone	Dolophine	II	4-6h	15-40	20 mg	10 mg
morphine sulfate	Roxanol	II	3-7h	2	60 mg	10 mg
nalbuphine	Nubain	N/A	3-6h	2-3	N/A	10 mg
oxycodone	Roxicodone	II	4-6h		30 mg	15 mg
oxymorphone	Numorphan	II	3-6h	2-3	6mg	1mg
pentazocine	Talwin	IV	2-3h	4-5	150 mg	30 mg
propoxyphene	Darvon	IV	4-6h	6-12	130 mg	N/A

a. Controlled substances schedule; b. ≈duration after single dose; c. dose is the amount that approximates the analgesic effect of 10 mg of morphine given SC or IM.
Adapted from Goodman and Gilman's, The Pharmacological Basis of Therapeutics, pg 497, 1990.

NARCOTICS

alfentanil *C2* [Alfenta] 5-20 mcg/kg IV increments
buprenorphine *C5* [Buprenex] 0.3 mg IV/IM q6h
butorphanol *C2* [Stadol, Stadol NS] 1 mg IV increments or 1-4 mg IM q3-4h, Nasal 1 spray (1 mg) then may repeat in 60-90 min if needed, then the 2 spray sequence may be repeated in 3-4h prn
codeine sulfate *C2* (Tab 15, 30, 60 mg) PO 15-60 mg q4-6h, MAX 360 mg/24h
codeine phosphate *C2* 0.5 mg/kg up to 60 mg IM q4-6h, MAX 360 mg/24h
dezocine [Dalgan] IV 2.5-10 mg q2-4h or IM 5-20 mg q3-6h MAX 120 mg/24h
fentanyl citrate *C2* [Sublimaze] IV increments of 2-3 mcg/kg up to 100 mcg 30-60min preop for premedication
fentanyl citrate Transmucosal System [Fentanyl Oralet] (Lozenges 100, 200, 300, 400 mcg) *Adults:* 2.5 to 5 mcg/kg (Max 400 mcg); Pt. To suck on unit- peak effect 20-30 mins. [Actiq] (Loz on stick 200, 400, 600, 800, 1200, 1600 mcg) Initial 200 mcg, may redose once per cancer pain episode★
fentanyl transdermal *C2* [Duragesic](patch 25, 50, 75, 100 µg/h) start at 25 µg/h patch q72h
hydromorphone *C2* [Dilaudid] (Tab 2,4 mg Supp 3 mg) PO/IM/SC 1-2 mg q4-6h, PR 1 q6-8h
levorphanol *C2* [Levo-Dromoran] (Tab 2mg) PO/SC 2-3 mg q6-8hprn
meperidine *C2* [Demerol] (Tab 50,100,Syp 50mg/5ml)IM/SC/PO 50-150 mg q3-4h prn (1-1.5mg/kg up to 150 mg)
methadone *C2* [Dolophine] (Tab 5, 10, Sol 5, 10 mg/5ml) PO/IM/SC 2.5-10 mg q3-4h
morphine sulfate *C2* [Duramorph] IV 2-10 mg/70kg
morphine sulfate *C2* [MSIR] (Tab & Cap 15, 30 mg; Sol 10 & 20 mg/5ml; Conc 20 mg/1ml) 5-30 mg q4h
morphine sulfate SR*C2* [MS Contin,Roxanol SR](Elx 10,20mg/5ml; Supp 5, 10, 20, 30 mg; Tab 15,30,60,100,200mg)PO 10-30mg q4-8h; PR 5-30 mg PR q 4 hrs ★
nalbuphine [Nubain] IV/IM 5-10 mg q3-6h
naloxone [Narcan] antagonist ET/SC/IM/IV 0.4-2.0 mg, Child- 0.1mg/kg
opium *C3* [Paregoric] (Liq 2 mg morphine equivalent/5ml) PO 5-10 ml 1-4 times a day
oxycodone *C2* [Roxicodone] (Tab 5 mg, Syp 5 mg/5ml) [OxyIR] (5 mg Cap) PO 5 mg q6h prn.
OxyContin *C2* [oxycodone controlled release] (tab 10, 20, 40 mg) 10 mg q12h titrate to pain relief or 240 mg/D
oxymorphone *C2* [Numorphan] SC/IM 1-1.5 mg q4-6h, IV 0.5 mg
pentazocine *C4* [Talwin] SC/IM/IV 30 mg q3-4h, MAX 360 mg/24h (SC may cause tissue injury)
pentazocine + naloxone *C4* [Talwin NX] (Tab 50/0.5 mg) PO 1-2 tabs q3-4h, MAX 12 tabs/24h

propoxyphene HCL *C4* [Darvon] (Tab 65 mg) PO 1 tab q4h, MAX propoxyphene 390 mg/24h
propoxyphene napsylate *C4* [Darvon-N] (Tab 100 mg) PO 1 tab q4h, MAX propoxyphene 600 mg/24h
sufentanil *C2* [Sufenta] IV use as directed with general anesthetic or epidural

NSAIDS (Nonsteroidal anti-inflammatories)
Arthrotec 50 [Tab diclofenac 50 mg + misoprostol 200 mcg] > *18 yrs use* 1 tab 2-4 times daily.
aspirin OTC [Bayer, Ecotrin] (Tab 65, 75, 81, 325, 500, 650 mg; Supp 60, 120, 325, 650 mg) PO/PR q4-6h
bromfenac [Duract] withdrawn from the market 1998
celecoxib [Celebrex] (Cap 100, 200 mg) *Osteoarthritis* 200 mg/day divided QD or BID; *Rheumatoid Arthritis* 100 to 200 mg twice a day★
diclofenac sodium [Voltaren] (Tab 25, 50, 75 mg) PO 50 mg TID/QID, 75 mg BID, MAX 200 mg/24h
diclofenac sodium [Voltaren XR] (Tab 100 mg) 1 tab QD-BID.
diclofenac potassium [Cataflam] (Tab 50 mg) PO 1 tab TID
diflunisal [Dolobid] (Tab 250, 500 mg) PO 1,000 mg initially then 500 mg bid
etodolac [Lodine, Lodine XL] (Tab 200, 300 mg; XL 500 mg) PO 200-400 mg q6-8h, MAX 1200 mg/24h; XL 1 tab QD
fenoprofen [Nalfon] (Tab 200, 300, 600 mg) PO 200-600 mg TID/QID, MAX 3200 mg/24h
flurbiprofen [Ansaid] (Tab 50, 100 mg) PO 200-300 mg/24h divided BID/TID/QID, MAX 300 mg/24h
ibuprofen [Advil, Medipren, Motrin, Nuprin, Rufen, Childrens Advil] (Tab 200, 300, 400, 600, 800 mg; Susp 100 mg/5ml) PO Peds 5-10 mg/kg q4-6h Max 40 mg/kg/D; Adults 300-800 mg QID
indomethacin [Indocin, Indocin SR] (Tab 25, 50, {SR 75 mg}; Susp 25 mg/5ml; Supp 50m g) PO/PR 25-50 mg TID, SR 1 tab QD/BID, MAX 200 mg/24h
ketoprofen [Orudis] (Tab 25, 50, 75 mg) PO 50-75 mg TID, MAX 300 mg/24h
ketoprofen [Oruvail] (Tab 200mg) PO 1 tab QD (not for initial therapy, for small, >75yrs of age or renal impaired)
ketorolac [Toradol] (Tab 10 mg; IM 30, 60 mg; IV) PO 10 mg q4-6h; IM load 30-60 mg then IM 15-30 mg q6h, MAX 150 mg 1st Day then 120 mg/D; IV 30 mg (15mg for elderly or renal dz) q6h; short term use only <5 days
meclofenamate [Meclomen] (Tab 50, 100 mg) PO 50 mg TID/QID, MAX 400 mg/24h
mefenamic acid [Ponstel] (Tab 250 mg) PO 500 mg initial then 250 mg QID, not to exceed 1 week.
Mepergan (Cap 50 mg meperidine/ 25 mg promethazine; Inj 25 mg meperidine/25 mg promethazine) 1 tab q 4-6 hrs; 1-2 ml IM/IV q 3-4 hrs.★
nabumetone [Relafen] (Tab 500, 750 mg) PO 1000 mg QD/BID, MAX 2000 mg/24h
naproxen [Naprosyn] (Tab 250, 375, 500 mg Susp 125 mg/5ml) PO 250-500 mg BID, MAX 1500 mg/24h
naproxen sodium [Aleve] OTC (Tab 220 mg) PO MAX 1 Tab q8-12h, 3 tabs/24h
naproxen sodium [Anaprox] (Tab 275, DS 550 mg) PO 275 mg TID/QID, or 550 mgDS PO BID. MAX 1.65g/24h
naproxen sodium (controlled release) [Naprelan] (Tab 375, 500 mg) PO 1-2 tabs QD; Acute Gout - 2-3 tabs day one, then 2 tabs QD until attains subsides.
oxaprozin [Daypro] (Tab 600 mg) PO 1-2 tabs QD, MAX 1800 mg/D in divided doses
piroxicam [Feldene] (Tab 10, 20 mg) PO 20 mg QD, MAX 20 mg/D
rofecoxib [Vioxx] (Tab 12.5, 25 mg; Susp 12.5, 25 mg/5ml) *Osteoarthritis* 12.5-25 mg QD; *acute pain or dysmenorhea* 50 mg PO QD (>5days not studied) ★
salsalate [Disalcid] (Tab 500, 750 mg; Caps 500 mg) PO 3000 mg/24h divided BID or TID
sulindac [Clinoril] (Tab 150, 200 mg) PO 150-200 mg BID, MAX 400 mg/24h
tolmetin [Tolectin] (Tab 200, DS 400, 600 mg) PO 200-600 mg TID, MAX 1800 mg/D
Vicoprofen *C3* [Tab hydrocodone 7.5 mg + ibuprofen 200 mg] >*16 yrs use* 1 tab q4-6 hrs PRN. Max 5 tabs/D

Miscellaneous
tramadol [Ultram] (Tab 50 mg) 50-100 mg q4-6h prn pain. MAX 400 mg/D. Centrally acting.

Analgesic Notes:

ECG
RATE: Normal 60-100 bpm. Find a complex that falls on 0.2s line (thick) then count the fifths of a second until the next complex, the first would be 300 bpm, then 150, 100, 75, 60, 50, 43, 37, 33, & 30 bpm. See back cover
RHYTHM: Normal PR interval < 0.20 sec., Normal QRS duration < 0.12 sec.
Normal Sinus Rhythm: P wave before each normal QRS, rate 60-100 bpm.
Sinus Bradycardia: P wave before each normal QRS, rate < 60 bpm.
Sinus Tachycardia: P wave before each normal QRS, rate > 100 bpm.
Atrial Fibrillation: no P wave, varying rhythm, normal QRS.
Premature Atrial Contraction: early abnormal P wave from ectopic foci, normal QRS.
Ventricular Premature Complex (VPC): wide QRS, no P wave, ectopic beat, compensatory pause. If R falls on T wave, beware of further dysrhythmia (R on T phenomenon).
Ventricular Tachycardia: > 4 VPC's in rapid succession.

WIDE QRS TACHYCARDIAS	
Findings that support VENTRICULAR TACHYCARDIA (VT)	Findings that support SUPRAVENTRICULAR TACH (SVT) with Aberrancy
MORPHOLOGY • Precordial leads-absence of RS or any with RS >100 msec • V_1- single peak, qR or R, QR or RS, wide r or slurred down stroke to late nadir- >60 msec • V_6- nadir >70 msec, rS, S or QS, QS or S >15mm deep **POLARITY** • positive or negative concordance • left axis deviation, axis in "no man's land" **DISSOCIATION** • fusion beats • early non-aberrant capture beats • independent P waves **QRS DURATION** >140 msec.	**MORPHOLOGY** • rSR' in V_1 • QRS in V_6 • Early nadir in V_1 • Same BBB in previous EKG • Onset with premature P wave • V Slowing or Termination with increased Vagal tone • Long-short cycle sequence

★Most likely VT if pt has CHD history!! ★Use precordial leads to monitor, confirm in multiple leads.
[1]Marriot, Henry J.L.: *Miscellaneous Electrocardiography*: Presentation NOV 17, 1993, pp 14-20. [2]*A Textbook of Cardiovascular Medicine*, 5th ed, E Braunwald (ed). Philadelphia, Saunders, 1997, pp 640-704. [3]*Circulation*. 1991;83:1649-1659.

Ventricular Flutter: 200-300 bpm, single ectopic focus, "Sine wave" appearance, usually goes to V-Fib.
Ventricular Fibrillation: totally irregular, no pattern, many ectopic foci.
PEA (Pulseless Electrical Activity): sinus rhythm without a pulse.
Asystole: no electrical activity.
Heart Blocks:
  Sinoatrial: conduction block for at least 1 beat.
  Atrioventricular: PR interval >0.20 sec
    First Degree AV: Normal P-QRS-T segment with increased PR interval.
    Second Degree Mobitz I (Wenckebach): PR interval progressively increases until a QRS is dropped.
                   Mobitz II: PR interval is fixed, more P waves then QRS, QRS is dropped.
    Third Degree: Total AV disassociation, PR varies, no pattern, independent of atrial and ventricular rate.
  Bundle Branch Blocks: Sudden onset often indicates impending MI. Cannot call MI by ECG with LBBB.
    RBBB: prolonged QRS, triphasic complexes- V1:rsR', delayed intrinsicoid deflection, V6: qRs.
    LBBB: prolonged QRS, monophasic complexes- V6: monophasic R; ST segment & T wave are opposite of QRS, delayed intrinsicoid deflection; similar to I & aVL. V1: monophasic QS with sharp down slope.
Left Anterior Hemiblock: normal QRS duration; left axis deviation > -45°; small Q in I & aVL; small R in II, III & aVF; late intrinsicoid deflection in aVL; deep S in II, III & aVF
Left Posterior Hemiblock: normal QRS duration; right axis deviation >110h; small R in I & aVL; small Q in II, III & aVF; late intrinsicoid deflection in aVF; deep S in I & aVL; no RVH; ↑ QRS voltage in limb leads.
Wolff-Parkinson White (WPW): Pre-excitation through the Accessory Bundle of Kent-premature excitation of the septum. Delta wave- decreased PR interval, increased QRS.

INTERVALS & COMPLEXES

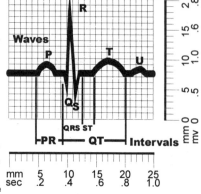

P Wave: Increased width- left atrial enlargement, diseased atria. Increased amplitude- atrial hypertrophy or dilation. Inversion- A-V junctional rhythm or ectopic atrial. Notching: left atrial involvement- mitral disease (P-mitrale) P wave wide & notched, taller in lead I than III. Peaking: right atrial overload (P-pulmonale) tall, pointed P > lead III than I. Absence: junctional rhythms, S-A block.

P-R Interval: Shortened: WPW syndrome, A-V junctional rhythm, some HTN, low atrial rhythm, Lown-Ganong-Levine syndrome, glycogen storage disease, Fabry's disease, pheochromocytoma. Prolonged: A-V block, normal variation, hyperthyroidism.

P-R Segment: displacement with acute pericarditis and atrial infarction.

QRS Complex: >0.12s: ventricular dysrhythmia or bundle branch block. Decreased Amplitude (<5mm average in limb leads): cardiac failure, pericardial effusion, coronary disease, amyloidosis, myxedema. Increased Amplitude: see Ventricular hypertrophy. Q wave: see infarction.

S-T Segment: Elevation: ischemia, transmural or subepicardial injury and occasional healthy young black men. Depression: subendocardial injury.

Q-T Duration: Should be < 1/2 the proceeding R-R interval during normal sinus rates. Prolonged (leads to R on T phenomenon): CHF, idiopathic, ischemic heart dz., rheumatic fever, myocarditis, hypokalemia with hypocalcemia, mitral valve prolapse, CVA. Shortened: hyperkalemia, hypercalcemia, digitalis toxicity.

T Wave: Normally- upright in I, II, V3-6; variable in III, aVL, aVF, V1-2; Inverted in aVR. Pointed: consider MI. Notching: children, pericarditis. Flat: obesity. Tall (>10mm): Hyperkalemia, CVA, myocardial ischemia.

U Wave: small wave following T wave with the same polarity: digitalis, quinidine, hypokalemia, thyrotoxicosis, epinephrine. Inverted: left anterior descending or left main coronary artery stenosis.

AXIS: If lead I and aVF are Positive then the axis is normal.

LEAD	+110	+90	+60	+30	0	-30	-45
I	–	=	+	+	+	+	+
II	+	+	+	+	+	–	–
III	+	+	+	=	–	–	–

HYPERTROPHY / ENLARGEMENT

Right Atrial Enlargement- P wave tall ≥2.5mm, pointed, lead III > I; frequently caused by pulmonary hypertension ("P-pulmonale") due to COPD, mitral valve stenosis or insufficiency and pulmonary emboli

Left Atrial Enlargement- (P-mitrale) P wave wide (≥0.12s) & notched (M shaped), taller in lead I than III; frequently due to mitral valve stenosis or insufficiency, systemic hypertension, hypertrophic cardiomyopathy

Left Ventricular Hypertrophy- (EKG diagnosis of LVH <60% sensitive and <95% specific) DDX- systemic hypertension, aortic stenosis or insufficiency, mitral insufficiency
- Simplified Criteria:
  - R wave: ≥ 20 mm in II, III or aVF; ≥ 12 mm in aVL; ≥ 25 mm in V5; ≥ 20 mm in V6
  - S wave: ≥ 20 mm in V1 or V2; Deepest S wave in V1 or V2, plus the tallest R wave in V5 or V6 ≥ 35 mm
  - LV Strain; ≥ 35 years old
- Estes Criteria- LVH if ≥ 5 points

R or S in limb lead ≥ 20 mm	3 pts	Left axis deviation of ≥15° ... 2
S in V1, V2 or V3 ≥ 25 mm	3	QRS ≥ 0.09s ... 1
ST-T changes	3	P terminal force in V1≥ 0.04s ... 3
With digitalis	1	Intrinsicoid deflection V5-6 ≥0.04s ... 1
R in V4,V5 or V6 ≥ 25 mm	3	

Right Ventricular Hypertrophy DDX- pulmonary valve disease, pulmonary hypertension, congenital heart disease. R/S ratio > in V1, V2; S/R ratio >1 in V5 & V6; right axis ≥ 110°; QRS < 0.12s

INFARCTION: The <u>THREE I's</u>:

<u>Ischemia:</u> inverted T wave. <u>Injury:</u> ST elevation- Acute; ST depression- subendocardial infarction, digitalis toxicity, positive stress test. <u>Infarction:</u> Significant Q wave: 1/3 QRS high & >1 mm wide. Insignificant Q wave: very small in I, II, V₅, V₆.

<u>Anterior wall MI:</u> Q waves & ST elevation in V₁-V₄ (Left anterior descending occlusion)
<u>Septal MI:</u> Q wave in V₁ & V₂
<u>Lateral MI:</u> Q waves & ST elevation in I & aVL (left circumflex occlusion)
<u>Inferior MI:</u> Q waves & ST elevation in II, III, aVF (right coronary artery occlusion)
<u>Posterior MI:</u> tall R & ST depression in V₁-V₃ (right coronary or left circumflex occlusion)

CARDIAC ENZYMES

<u>LDH</u>
1-Heart, RBC's, renal cortex, pancreas
2-RBC's, heart, spleen, lung, thyroid
3-Lung, spleen, LN, adrenals, thyroid
4-Lung, adrenals, skeletal muscle
5-Liver, skeletal muscle, WBC

<u>CK</u>
CK-MM: skeletal muscle 100%, cardiac muscle 85%
CK-MB: cardiac 15-20%
CK-BB: brain, lung, smooth muscle

LDH Isoenzyme Patterns:
LDH1 / LDH2 flip = AMI, RBC hemolysis.
Isolated elevation of LDH5 = Liver congestion/ inflammation.
Elevated LDH1 and LDH5 = MI with Right heart failure and liver congestion.

CARDIAC MARKER ELEVATION	Onset (hr)	Peak (hr)	Normalizes (days)
Cardiac specific troponin (cTnT)	1-2		10-14
Cardiac specific troponin I (cTnI)	1-2		7-10
Myoglobin	1-2		1
Total CK	4-8	12-24	2-3
CK-MB	4-8	12-24	1.5-3
Total LDH	8-12	72-144	10-14
LDH1/LDH2 flip	14	48-72	7-14
Total AST	6-52	20-48	5-9

ACUTE MI DIAGNOSIS	Sensitivity (%)	Specificity (%)
ECG	+(63-73)	++++(100)
Cardiac specific troponin (cTnT)	+++++	++++
Cardiac specific troponin I (cTnI)	+++++	++++
Myoglobin	+++	+
Total CK	+++++(98)	++(65)
CK-MB	+++++(100)	+++++(98)
Total LDH	+++++(98-100)	++(70)
LDH 1/LDH2 flip	+++(80)	++++(94-97)
Serum AST	+++++(98)	++(71)

ECG PATTERNS

Digitalis Toxicity: VPC's, Ventricular Tachycardia, Ventricular Fibrillation, Atrial Fibrillation, ↓ ST segment.
Hypercalcemia: QT interval short; SX: N/V, headache, confusion, anorexia, abdominal pain, polyuria, polydipsia.
Hypocalcemia: QT prolongation; SX: tetany, tremors, seizures, muscle spasms, bronchospasm, ↓Cardiac output
Hyperkalemia: typical ECG progression: thin peaked T waves→ depressed ST segment→ increased PR→ flat P waves→ increased QRS→ sine wave pattern- "Fatal ventricular dysrhythmias" (when K⁺>6.5 mmol/L), SX: confusion, muscle weakness.
Hypokalemia: PAC's, VPC's, flat T wave, U wave, depressed ST, SX: headache, dizziness, muscle weakness.
Hypermagnesemia: peaked T wave, bradycardia, hypotension; SX: muscle weakness, lethargy, apnea.
Hypomagnesemia: flat T wave, ST depression, QT prolongation, SX: confusion, seizures, coma, lethargy.
Pericardial effusion: electrical alternans
Pericarditis: precordial ST segment elevation and PR depression.
Pulmonary Emboli: Sinus tachycardia, Non-specific ST changes, S₁ Q₃ ⊥₃ pattern (large S wave in lead I, Q wave in lead III, inverted T wave in lead III).
ST elevation without ischemia: early repolarization (J point), pericarditis, left ventricular aneurysm.
Ventricular Aneurysm: elevated ST segment- does not return to baseline with time.
Ventricular Strain: depressed ST segment in V₁-₂ for right and V₅-₆ for left Ventricular Strain.

BLEEDING FACTORS

<u>Extrinsic Clotting System</u>: Tissue thromboplastin, & factors V, VII, X. Monitored with Prothrombin time (PT).

<u>Intrinsic Clotting System</u>: Factors I, II, V, VIII, IX, X, XI, XII. Monitor with PTT.

<u>Partial Thromboplastin Time, Activated</u> (PTT): Test for all clotting factors except for VII. DDX of ↑ PTT: Vit. K def., liver disease, DIC, factor I, II, V, VIII, IX, X, XI, & XII deficiency, nephrotic syndrome, dysproteinemias.

<u>International Normalization Ratio(INR)</u>: DDX of ↑ INR: warfarin, heparin, DIC, cirrhosis, Vit K deficiency, factor I, II, V, VII, X def. INR replaces Prothrombin time allowing for variations between lots of thromboplastin.

<u>Heparin</u>: Activates antithrombin III. Protamine sulfate reverses heparin effects. Therapeutic- 1.5-2.0 times control.

<u>Warfarin</u>: reduces the synthesis of Vit. K dependent clotting Factors (VII, IX, X, II; t½ 6, 24, 36, 50h, respectively). Factor VII is affected first prolonging the INR in 8-12h, although maximum anticoagulation is not achieved for 3-5 days when all the Vit K dependent factors are depleted.

Therapeutic- INR of 2.0-3.0 for: prophylaxis of venous thrombosis (high risk surgery), treatment of venous thrombosis, treatment of pulmonary embolism, tissue heart valves, acute MI, valvular heart disease, atrial fibrillation. *INR of 2.5-3.5* for: mechanical heart valves.

CHEST PAIN

DIFFERENTIAL DIAGNOSES: Cardiac: Myocardial infarction, angina, valvular disease, aortic dissection or aneurysm, IHSS, pericarditis, neoplasm. GI: PUD, esophagitis, esophageal spasm, Mallory-Weiss syndrome, carcinoma, Zenker's diverticulum, cholecystitis, pancreatitis. Pulmonary: Pleuritis, bronchitis, pneumonia, neoplasm, pulmonary embolus, pneumothorax, trauma. Musculoskeletal: Costochondritis, muscle spasm, trauma, intercostal myositis, thoracic outlet syndrome. Misc.: Herpes Zoster, Tabes dorsalis, breast lesions.

WORK-UP History: MOST IMPORTANT- Onset, duration, severity, quality, frequency, palliative measures, previous episodes, cardiac risk factors, associated symptoms, trauma Physical Exam: Vital signs, diaphoresis, vision, equal radial pulse, attempt to reproduce pain, auscultate for gallops/ rubs/ murmurs, left or right ventricular heave, auscultate lungs, abdomen for tenderness/ guarding/ rebound. Labs: ECG, Chest X-ray, ABG, serial cardiac enzymes, others as indicated by working diagnosis.

TREATMENT Oxygen 6-10 L via Face Mask. If patient is a CO_2 retainer, use caution, 2 L via nasal cannula. Nitroglycerin 0.4 mg SL q5 min (if systolic BP > 90 mmHg). If pain persists after three doses of NTG, Morphine 10 mg in 9 ml NS given in 2-4 mg doses IV if systolic BP >90 mmHg, until pain is relieved. Aspirin, NTG IV, thrombolytics or PTCA if indicated. Treat specific etiology as recommended in current literature.

See ACLS algorithm for myocardial infarction.

<u>ALWAYS</u>: Get a Good History. Get Vitals before treating. Get Old ECG to compare to present ECG.

KILLIP CLASSIFICATION OF HEART FAILURE IN ACUTE MYOCARDIAL INFARCTION

Class I   No signs of heart failure. Mortality < 5%.

Class II   Mild or moderate heart failure: rales can be heard over as much as 50 percent of both lung fields

Class III   Pulmonary edema: rales can be heard over more than half of both lung fields

Class IV   Cardiogenic shock: blood pressure < 90 mmHg; signs of inadequate peripheral perfusion are evident, including ↓ urine flow, cold & clammy skin, cyanosis, mental obtundation. Mortality 80%.

CLINICAL & HEMODYNAMIC CLASSES OF AMI*	Cardiac Index	PCWP	BP
I No pulmonary congestion or peripheral hypoperfusion	2.7 ± 0.5	≤ 12	normal
Rx : IV Nitro to modify mortality, infarct size, & pain.			
II Isolated pulmonary congestion	> 3.0	< 12	↑
Rx: IV Nitro, diuretics (decrease preload), morphine.			
III Isolated peripheral hypotension	≤ 2.7	≤ 9	↓
Rx: Careful hydration (increased PCWP to approx. 18)			
IV Both pulmonary congestion & peripheral hypotension			
Mild LV failure	≤ 2.5	>18 ≤ 22	normal
Severe LV failure	≤ 1.8	≥ 22	↑ ↓
Rx: Combined use of Dopamine & Dobutamine			
or Amrinone), consider Intraaortic Balloon Pump			
V Cardiogenic shock	≤ 1.8	≥ 18	↓
Rx: PTCA or CABG and circulatory support			
VI Shock secondary to right ventricular infarction	≤ 1.8	≤ 18	↓
Rx: support circulatory volume and inotropics			

*Data from J. Am. Coll. Cardiol. 16:249, 1990

NEW YORK HEART CLASSIFICATION OF CARDIOVASCULAR DISEASE
- Etiology: include both structural & functional disturbances (ex: Coronary atherosclerosis)
- Anatomy: lesions of heart & great vessels (ex: 90% cross-sectional obstruction of LAD; normal heart size)
- Physiology: all physiologic disturbances, include CCS class of angina heart failure (ex: Unstable angina pectoris (recent onset- Class 2 CCS). No heart failure, good contractility; normal sinus rhythm)
- Cardiac Status: total assessment of the etiologic, anatomic, & physiologic diagnosis.
  Class 1 - Not compromised; Class 2 - Slightly compromised; Class 3 - Moderately compromised
  Class 4 - Severely compromised
- Prognosis: assessment of potential effects of optimal current medical & surgical therapies
  Class 1 - Good; Class 2 - Good with therapy; Class 3 - Fair with therapy; Class 4 - Guarded despite therapy
- Specific Recommendations: Further diagnostic procedures; limitation of physical activity; medical or surgical correction; antibiotics; dietary restrictions; cardiac medications; etc.

CANADIAN CARDIOVASCULAR CLASSIFICATION OF ANGINA SEVERITY (CCS)

Class I	Angina with strenuous or prolonged exertion; not ordinary activity (e.g., climbing stairs or walking)
Class II	Mild limitation of ordinary activity; (climbing stairs rapidly or after meals, walking uphill, walking after meals, or in wind, or under emotional stress, or only during few hs after waking in morning. Walking > 2 level blocks & climbing > 1 flight of stairs at normal pace & conditions).
Class III	Marked limitation of ordinary physical activity;(walking 1-2 blocks or climbing 1 flight of stairs)
Class IV	Unable to carry on any physical activity without discomfort (May be present at rest).

AMERICAN SOCIETY of ANESTHESIOLOGISTS PREOPERATIVE PATIENT CLASSIFICATION
(NOTE: Negative predictive value far exceeds Positive predictive value)48 hour Mortality

I	Healthy patient	0.07%
II	Mild systemic disease	0.24%
III	Severe systemic disease, limits activity but is not incapacitating	1.4%
IV	Incapacitating systemic disease which is a constant threat to life	7.5%
V	Moribund, not expected to survive 24 hr. with or without operation	8.1%
E	Add to class if an emergency	Doubles the Risk

CARDIAC RISK INDEX(CRI)(Goldman Criteria[1,2]) Points: Goldman   Detsky   Larsen

		Goldman	Detsky	Larsen
History	• Age >70 years	5	5	
	• MI within 3 months		11	
	> 3 months ago and/or angina		3	
	within 6 months	10		5
	> 6 months ago	5		
	• Angina: Unstable (in the last 6 mo)	10		
	CCS class III/[IV]		10 [20]	
Physical examination	• S3 gallop or JVD	11		
	• Hx of pulmonary edema [or in the last wk]	5 [10]	8	
	persistent pulmonary congestion		12	
	• Hx of heart failure		4	
	• Aortic stenosis*(Important) †(suspected critical)	3*	20†	
ECG	• Rhythm other than sinus or PAC's on last ECG	7	5	
	• Documented PVCs *(>5/min) †(>7/min)	7*	5†	
General status		3	5	
	• PaO2< 60, PaCO2>50mmHg, K+ <3, HCO3< 20,BUN>50,Creatinine > 3.0,↑ SGOT, chronic liver dz, or bedridden from noncardiac causes			
	• Serum Creatinine >0.13 mmol/L⁻¹		2	
	• Diabetes		3	
Operation:	• Intraperitoneal, intrathoracic, *(or aortic)	3*	3	
	• Aortic			5
	• Emergency	4	10	3
	TOTAL POSSIBLE POINTS	53	80	

Predicted Risk of Perioperative Complications: MI, cardiogenic pulmonary edema, VT, VF, cardiac death					
CRI	Goldman		Larsen		Detsky	
Class	Points Minor surgery	High-risk†	Points		Points	
I	0-5	0.3%	3%	0-5	0.5%	0-15	0.4%
II	6-12	1.0%	10%	6-7	3.8%	16-30	4%
III	13-25	3%	30%	8-14	11%	>30	15%
IV	≥26	15%	80%	>15	58%		

†known CAD, abd aortic surgery or other high risk. [1]Modified from Goldman, L., et al.: Multifactorial Index of Cardiac Risk in Non-Cardiac Surgical Procedures. *N. Engl. J. Med.* 297:845,1977.[2]*Heart Disease: A Textbook of Cardiovascular Medicine*, 5th ed, E Braunwald (ed). Philadelphia, Saunders, 1997, pp 108-152

EXERCISE STRESS TESTING (GST):[1,2] Indications for GXT based on the ACC/AHA classification (•- testing to diagnose CAD; + for Risk assessment and prognosis; ♥ after MI; ✚ asymptomatic persons without known CAD; ⊗ evaluation of patients with valvular heart disease; ⊃ before & after revascularization; ⌇ investigation of dysrhythmias)

CLASS I (conditions with evidence and/or general agreement that the procedure is useful and effective)
- •Adults with an intermediate pretest probability of CAD
- +Patients undergoing initial evaluation with suspected or known CAD; Patients with suspected or known CAD previously evaluated with significant change in clinical status
- ♥Before discharge, early after discharge or late after discharge for prognostic assessment, activity prescription, evaluation of medical therapy
- ⊃To demonstrate ischemia before revascularization; evaluation of recurrent symptoms after revascularization
- ⌇evaluation for settings in patients with rate-adaptive pacemakers

CLASS II (conditions with conflicting evidence or a divergence of opinion about the usefulness /efficacy)
IIa: (weight of evidence/opinion is in favor of usefulness/efficacy)
- •Patients with vasospastic angina
- ♥, ⊃after discharge for activity counseling and/or exercise training as part of cardiac rehabilitation after revascularization.
- ⌇To diagnose out and evaluate therapy for exercise induced arrhythmia

IIb (usefulness/efficacy is less well established by evidence/opinion)
- •Patients with a high or low pretest probability of CAD by age, symptoms and gender; Patients with less than 1 mm of baseline ST depression and taking digoxin; Patients with EKG criteria for LVH and less than 1 mm of baseline ST depression
- +Patients with: preexcitation syndrome, electronically paced ventricular rhythm, greater than 1 mm of resting ST depression, complete LBBB; Patients with a stable clinical course who undergo periodic monitoring to guide treatment.
- ♥Before discharge after cardiac catheterization demonstrating borderline severity; Patients with: preexcitation syndrome, electronically paced ventricular rhythm, greater than 1 mm of resting ST depression, digoxin, complete LBBB; Patients with a stable clinical course who undergo periodic monitoring to guide treatment.
- ✚ evaluation of patients with multiple risk factors; ♂ >40 or ♀ >50 years who plan to start a vigorous exercise program, occupations in which impairment might impact public safety or patients high risk for CAD
- ⊗evaluation of exercise capacity of patients with valvular heart disease
- ⊃detection of restenosis in high risk asymptomatic patients after angioplasty; periodic monitoring of high risk asymptomatic patients for restenosis or disease progression
- ⌇Evaluation of isolated VEB in middle-aged persons without other evidence of CAD

CLASS III (conditions with evidence and/or general agreement that the procedure is not useful or effective and in some cases may be harmful)
- •Patients with: preexcitation syndrome, electronically paced ventricular rhythm, greater than 1 mm of resting ST depression, complete LBBB; Patients with documented myocardial infarction or prior coronary angiography demonstrating significant disease have an established diagnosis of CAD
- +♥Patients with severe comorbidity likely to limit life expectancy and/or candidacy for revascularization
- ✚ Routine screening of asymptomatic men or women
- ⊗diagnosis of CAD in patients with valvular disease
- ⊃Periodic monitoring of asymptomatic patients after PTCA or CABG without specific indications; localization of ischemia to determine the site of intervention.
- ⌇Evaluation of isolated VEB in young persons without other evidence of CAD

CONTRAINDICATIONS TO TESTING: symptomatic severe aortic stenosis, uncontrolled symptomatic heart failure, unstable angina (not previously stabilized by medical therapy, ACUTE MI within 2 days, acute pulmonary embolism or infarction, uncontrolled symptomatic cardiac arrhythmias, acute aortic dissection, acute myocarditis or pericarditis.

RELATIVE CONTRAINDICATIONS- moderate stenotic valvular heart disease, left main coronary artery stenosis, electrolyte abnormalities, severe arterial hypertension, tachyarrhythmias or bradyarrhythmias, physical or mental impairment leading to the inability to exercise adequately, high grade atrioventricular block, hypertrophic cardiomyopathy and other outflow tract obstruction.

ADEQUATE TEST- good double product ≥20,000(HR x Systolic BP, correlates with myocardial O_2 demand). Interpretation of the exercise test should include exercise capacity and hemodynamic, clinical, and electrocardiographic response. The most important electrocardiographic findings are ST depression and elevation. ECG positive- ≥1 mm of horizontal or down sloping ST-segment depression or elevation for at least 60 to 80 milliseconds after the J point (end of the QRS complex). Clinically positive-The occurrence of ischemic chest pain consistent with angina, especially if it is the reason for termination of the test. Good prognosis if- negative test or if test is positive after stage 3 of Bruce protocol or after HR > 160 bpm.

[1] *Circulation.* 1997;96:345-354. [2]Chaitman BR: Exercise Stress testing, in *Heart Disease: A Textbook of Cardiovascular Medicine,* 5th ed, E Braunwald (ed). Philadelphia, Saunders, 1997, pp 153-162

CARDIAC CONDITIONS ASSOCIATED WITH ENDOCARDITIS [1]

Endocarditis prophylaxis recommended	
High risk category:	Moderate risk category
•Prosthetic cardiac valves •Previous bacterial endocarditis •Complex cyanotic congenital heart disease •Surgical construction of pulmonary shunts or conduits	•Other congenital cardiac malformations (other than listed above or below) •Acquired valve dysfunction (i.e. rheumatic heart disease) •Hypertrophic cardiomyopathy •MVP with regurgitation and/or thickened leaflets[1]

Endocarditis prophylaxis **not** recommended	
Negligible risk category (no greater risk than general population)	
•Isolated secundum atrial septal defect •Surgical repair of ASD, ventricular septal defect, or patent ductus arteriosus (without defect beyond 6 months) •Previous coronary artery bypass graft surgery •Mitral valve prolapse without valvar dysfunction[1]	•Physiologic, functional or innocent heart murmurs* •Previous Kawasaki disease without valvar dysfunction •Previous Rheumatic fever without valvar dysfunction •Cardiac pacemakers and implanted defibrillators

*Anterior mitral valve thickening in men older than 45 years with MVP, without a consistent systolic murmur, may warrant prophylaxis even in the absence of resting regurgitation. Myxomatous mitral valve degeneration with regurgitation is an indication for antibiotic prophylaxis in any age group.

ENDOCARDITIS PROPHYLAXIS FOR DENTAL PROCEDURES [1]

Endocarditis prophylaxis recommended- high and moderate risk cardiac conditions	
•Dental extractions •Periodontal procedures (surgery, scaling and root planing, probing and recall maintenance •Dental implant placement and reimplantation of avulsed teeth •Root canal instrumentation or surgery beyond the apex	•Subgingival placement of antibiotic fibers or strips •Initial placement of orthodontic bands but not brackets •Intraligamentary local anesthetic injections •Prophylactic cleaning of teeth or implants where bleeding is anticipated

Endocarditis prophylaxis **not** recommended	
•Restorative dentistry † (operative and prosthodontic) with or without retraction cord ‡ •Local anesthetic injections(non-intraligamentary) •Intracanal endodontic treatment; post placement and buildup •Placement of rubber dams	•Postoperative suture removal •Placement of removable prosthodontic or orthodontic appliances •Taking of oral impressions •Fluoride treatments •Taking of oral radiographs •Orthodontic appliance adjustment •Shedding of primary teeth

*Prophylaxis is recommended for patients with high- and moderate-risk cardiac conditions.
† This includes restoration of decayed teeth (filling cavities) and replacement of missing teeth.
‡ Clinical judgment may indicate antibiotic use in selected circumstances that may create significant bleeding.

OTHER PROCEDURES AND ENDOCARDITIS PROPHYLAXIS

Endocarditis prophylaxis recommended	
•<u>Gastrointestinal tract</u>* Sclerotherapy for esophageal varices Esophageal stricture dilation Endoscopic retrograde cholangiography with biliary obstruction Biliary tract surgery Surgical operations involving intestinal mucosa	•<u>Respiratory tract</u> Tonsillectomy and/or adenoidectomy Surgical operations involving respiratory mucosa Bronchoscopy with a rigid bronchoscope •<u>Genitourinary tract</u> Prostatic surgery, Cystoscopy, Urethral dilation •<u>Infected Tissues</u> procedures involving infected tissue (i.e. I&D)

[1]data from AMA recommendations, *JAMA.* 1997;277:1794-1801

Endocarditis prophylaxis **not** recommended [1]	

•Gastrointestinal tract
Transesophageal echocardiography †
  Endoscopy with or without gastrointestinal
Biopsy †
•Genitourinary tract
  Vaginal hysterectomy †
  Vaginal delivery †
  Cesarean section
  In uninfected tissue: Urethral catheterization,
  Uterine dilatation and curettage, Therapeutic
  Abortion, Sterilization procedures, Insertion or
  Removal of intrauterine devices
	•Respiratory tract
	  Endotracheal intubation
	  Bronchoscopy with a flexible bronchoscope,
	  With or without biopsy †
	  Tympanostomy tube insertion
	•Other
	  Cardiac catheterization, including balloon
	  Angioplasty
	  Implanted cardiac pacemakers, implanted
	  Defibrillators, and coronary stents
	  Incision or biopsy of surgically scrubbed skin
	  Circumcision

*Prophylaxis is recommended for high-risk patients; it is optional for medium-risk patients.
† Prophylaxis is optional for high-risk patients.

PROPHYLACTIC REGIMENS FOR DENTAL, ORAL, RESPIRATORY TRACT, OR ESOPHAGEAL PROCEDURES [1]		
Situation	Agent	Regimen
Standard general prophylaxis	Amoxicillin	Adults: 2.0 g; children: 50 mg/kg orally 1 h before procedure
Unable to take oral medications	Ampicillin	Adults: 2.0 g IM or IV; children: 50 mg/kg IM or IV within 30 min before procedure
Allergic to penicillin	Clindamycin	Adults: 600 mg; children: 20 mg/kg orally 1 h before procedure
	Cephalexin † or cefadroxil †	Adults: 2.0 g; children: 50 mg/kg orally 1 h before procedure
	Azithromycin or clarithromycin	Adults: 500 mg; children: 15 mg/kg orally 1 h before procedure
Allergic to penicillin and unable to take oral medications	Clindamycin or Cefazolin †	Adults: 600 mg; children: 20 mg/kg IV within 30 min before procedure Adults: 1.0 g; children: 25 mg/kg IM or IV within 30 min before procedure

*Total children's dose should not exceed adult dose. † Cephalosporins should not be used in individuals with immediate-type hypersensitivity reaction (urticaria, angioedema, or anaphylaxis) to penicillins.

Prophylactic Regimens for Genitourinary/Gastrointestinal (Except esophageal-see above) Procedures		
Situation	Agent	Regimen
High-risk patients	Ampicillin and gentamicin	Adults: ampicillin 2.0 g IM or IV plus gentamicin 1.5 mg/kg (not to exceed 120 mg) within 30 min of starting procedure; 6 h later, ampicillin 1 g IM/IV or amoxicillin 1 g orally Children: ampicillin 50 mg/kg IM or IV (not to exceed 2.0 g) plus gentamicin 1.5 mg/kg within 30 min of starting the procedure; 6 h later, ampicillin 25 mg/kg IM/IV or amoxicillin 25 mg/kg orally
High-risk patients Allergic to penicillin	Vancomycin and gentamicin	Adults: vancomycin 1.0 g IV over 1-2 h plus gentamicin 1.5 mg/kg IV/IM (not to exceed 120 mg); complete injection/infusion within 30 min of starting procedure Children: vancomycin 20 mg/kg IV over 1-2 h plus gentamicin 1.5 mg/kg IV/IM; complete injection/infusion within 30 min of starting procedure
Moderate-risk patients	Amoxicillin or ampicillin	Adults: amoxicillin 2.0 g orally 1 h before procedure, or ampicillin 2.0 g IM/IV within 30 min of starting procedure Children: amoxicillin 50 mg/kg orally 1 h before procedure, or ampicillin 50 mg/kg IM/IV within 30 min of starting procedure
Moderate-risk patients Allergic to penicillin	Vancomycin	Adults: vancomycin 1.0 g IV over 1-2 h complete infusion within 30 min of starting procedure Children: vancomycin 20 mg/kg IV over 1-2 h; complete infusion within 30 min of starting procedure

*Total children's dose should not exceed adult dose. † no second dose of gentamicin or vancomycin is recommended

[1]data from AMA recommendations, *JAMA*. 1997;277:1794-1801

JONES CRITERIA for Rheumatic Fever (American Heart Association, 1992)	
Major Criteria	**Minor Criteria**
•Carditis •Migratory Polyarthritis •Sydenham's Chorea •Erythema marginatum •Subcutaneous nodules	Clinical: •arthralgia •fever Lab: •↑ESR •↑CRP •Prolonged PR interval •↑ acute phase reactants
Plus: Supporting Evidence of Antecedent group A Strep Infection: Positive throat culture or Rapid Strep antigen test, Elevated or rising Streptococcal antibody titer.	
• If supported by evidence of antecedent group A strep infection, then the presence of 2 major OR of 1 major & 2 minor criteria indicate a high probability of acute rheumatic fever.	

HEAST SOUNDS AND MURMURS

S_1: ↑Intensity – MVP, ↑HR, MS, ↓PR interval, Ebstein anomaly. ↓Intensity- LV dysfunction, LBBB, MR, ↑PR interval, calcified mitral valve

S_2: Normal splits on inspiration (A_2-P_2) and single sound on expiration. Reversed splitting (Paradoxical)- LBBB, AS, PDA, RV ectopy, RV pacing. Fixed splitting- ASD. Persistent or wide splitting- MR, PS, RBBB, VSD, LV ectopy

Murmurs: Continuous-PDA, AV fistula, pregnancy(Mammary souffle'),Tetralogy of Fallot. Holosystolic: TR, MR, VSD

Dynamic Auscultation	AS	MR	IHSS	TR	AR	MS	TS	PS	VSD	TOF	Austin-Flint	AV fistula
Inspiration ↑ venous return (VR)				↑			↑	↑				
Valsalva ↓VR, ↓ Stroke Vol (SV)	↓	↓	↑	↓	↓	↓	↓	↓				
Squatting ↑VR, ↑SVR, ↑SV	↑	↑	↓		↑	↑	↑	↑	↑	↑		
Supine ↑VR	↑	↑	↓	↑			↑	↑				
Isometric exercise ↑SVR, ↑HR, ↑CO, ↑MAP, ↑heart size	↓	↑	↓	↑	↑			↑				
Amyl nitrates ↓SVR	↑	↓	↑	↑	↓					↑	↓	

VALVULAR HEART DISEASE

Aortic Stenosis- DDX: congenital (bicuspid valve most common), rheumatic fever or degeneration (elderly). Symptoms-chest pain (2-5y survival), syncope (2-5y survival) & heart failure (2y life expectancy). Crescendo-decrescendo systolic murmur, pulsus tardus & LVH. DX: echo- LV thickness & EF, # of leaflets, doppler gradient. Left heart cath- normal orifice 2.5-3 cm² (mild stenosis 0.75-1.5, moderate <0.75, severe <0.5) & gradient measurement. Surgery if gradient > 50mmHg or area <.08 cm². Antibiotic prophylaxis see below.

HYPERTENSION
MEDICAL HISTORY

Review of Systems: Previous history of hypertension or use of cardiac medications. Onset and level of elevated blood pressure. Patient history of symptoms of CHD, heart failure, diabetes mellitus, renal disease, cerebrovascular disease, dyslipidemia, chest pain or discomfort, palpitations, tachycardia, edema, heart murmur, irregular rhythm, exertional dyspnea, cough, cyanosis, ascites, intermittent claudication, thrombophlebitis, rheumatic fever, sexual dysfunction, family history of premature CHD. Recent weight changes.

Lifestyle: smoking or other tobacco; exercise type, frequency and duration; Diet: intake of sodium, saturated fat, alcohol and caffeine; Illicit drug use; psychosocial and environmental factors.

Current medications: Prescription names, strength and frequency, including over the counter and natural remedies.

PHYSICAL EXAM

Blood pressure measurements 2 or more times and confirmed in contralateral arm (use highest reading). Measure height, waist circumference and weight. Funduscopic exam for retinopathy. Neck: bruits and thyroid. Cardiac: rate, murmurs, gallops, rubs, clicks, ventricular heaves or other visible precordial movements. Evaluation of the apical impulse and the symmetry and quality of the carotid, radial, femoral, posterior tibial and dorsalis pedis pulses. Lungs: rales and rhonchi. Abdomen: bruits, masses, kidney size, aortic pulsation. Neurological exam for deficits.

LABS AND OTHER TESTS

CBC, lytes, glucose, creatinine, lipid profile, urinalysis, and 12-lead electrocardiogram. Consider microalbumin, 24 hour urinary creatinine & protein, uric acid, thyroid stimulating hormone, glycated hemoglobin, echocardiogram, arterial ultrasounds, ankle/brachial index, plasma renin activity/urinary sodium determination.

Classification of Blood Pressure for Adults (≥18 years)*		
Category	Diastolic	Systolic
Optimal	<80	<120
Normal	<85	<130
High Normal	85-89	130-139
Hypertension†		
Stage I (Mild)	90-99	140-159
Stage II (Moderate)	100-109	160-179
Stage III (Severe)	≥110	≥180
Follow-up recommendations based on the Initial BP Measurement §		
Normal	Recheck within 2 years	
High Normal	Recheck within 1 year	
Stage I (Mild)	Recheck within 2 months	
Stage II (Moderate)	Evaluate or refer within 1 month	
Stage III (Severe)	Evaluate or refer immediately or refer within 1 week depending on patient's condition	

*JNC 6th Report, *Arch Intern Med.* 1997;157:2413-2446. When the diastolic and systolic blood pressures fall into different categories, the higher category should be selected. †Based on the average of 2 or more readings after the initial high reading. §Modify follow-up interval based on specific clinical factors (i.e. other cardiac risk factors, target organ disease, and history of previous blood pressure measurements).

DIFFERENTIAL DIAGNOSIS

ESSENTIAL HTN >90% of patients with HTN have no identifiable cause.

SECONDARY HTN- *Consider if: Age, H&P, stage of HTN, and labs suggest; Poorly responsive to drug therapy; sudden increase in blood pressure; Sudden onset of HTN; Stage 3 HTN.*

Renovascular- Most common cause of 2° HTN. Hematuria, flank pain, abrupt onset of severe uncontrolled HTN, abdominal bruits (over renal areas or diastolic component) retinopathy and papilledema usually present. Fibro-muscular hyperplasia (female, beading effect) and atherosclerotic renal disease (male- proximal narrowing) are the two most common causes. **DX:** peripheral venous renin increased, rapid sequence IV pyelogram, arteriogram

Primary Aldosteronism (Conn's Syndrome): Low renin hypertension from excess mineralocorticoid. Proximal muscle weakness, fatigue, cramps, and tetany from hypokalemia induced metabolic alkalosis. Edema is not a feature, because of the escape mechanism of Na^+. **DX:** Plasma Renin activity (renin suppressed even after Lasix), 24 hr U_K^+> 50 mmol/24 hr, 24 hr Urine Aldosterone on high NA^+ diet (to exclude 2° Aldosterone release), serum electrolytes, plasma aldosterone, precursor steroids. Confirm: 2 L Saline IV over 4 hr (baseline and post plasma aldosterone levels), Captopril test, mineralocorticoid infusion, Spironolactone therapy.

Secondary Aldosteronism: increased Aldosterone secondary to increased Renin activity in CHF, Cirrhosis, Nephrotic syndrome or any volume depleted state.

Pheochromocytoma: Increased release of catecholamines. Triad of headache, perspiration and palpitations. Orthostatic hypotension, normotensive during sleep, increased 24-hr urine metanephrine, clonidine suppression.

Cushing's Syndrome: Thin skin with purple striae, truncal obesity, muscle atrophy, increased 24 hr urine free cortisol, abnormal low dose dexamethasone suppression test and high dose dexamethasone suppression test.

Bartter's Syndrome: Rare Disease. Most commonly found in children. Hypokalemic metabolic alkalosis, hyperreninemia, hyperaldosteronism.

Liddle's Syndrome: Rare disease of tubular transport. Resembles Primary aldosteronism, except plasma aldosterone is normal. Responds to spironolactone. The Distal Tubules behave as if been exposed to aldosterone. May represent exaggerated response to normal levels of mineralocorticoid.

RISK STRATIFICATION

Risk Group	Blood Pressure Stages		
	High-normal	Stage 1	Stage 2 & 3
A- No RF*, TOD/CCD[†]	Lifestyle modification[‡]	Lifestyle modification[‡] up to 12 months	Drug Therapy[§]
B- ≥1 RF* (other than DM) No TOD/CCD[†]	Lifestyle modification[‡]	Lifestyle modification[‡] up to 6 months	Drug Therapy
C-TOD/CCD[†] and /or DIABETES MELLITUS, with/without other RF*	Drug Therapy[§]	Drug Therapy[§]	Drug Therapy

*RF= Risk Factors, [†]TOD/CCD= Target Organ Disease/Clinical Cardiovascular Disease; see table below.
[‡]Lifestyle modification should also be adjunctive therapy for all patients on drug therapy. [§]Drug Therapy for patients with diabetes, heart failure or renal insufficiency.

MAJOR RISK FACTORS

Smoking	Gender- men and postmenopausal women
Diabetes	FMH of CHD □<55 or □<65 years
Dyslipidemia	Age > 60 years
Target Organ Disease / Clinical Cardiovascular Disease	
Heart Diseases:	Stroke or TIA
LVH	Nephropathy
Angina or prior MI	Retinopathy
Heart Failure	Peripheral artery disease
Prior coronary revascularization	

TREATMENT
LIFESTYLE MODIFICATION
- Weight loss if overweight
- Limit alcohol intake
- Increase aerobic activity – 30-45 minutes 5-7 days a week
- Maintain adequate intake of dietary potassium (50-90 mmol/d), calcium and magnesium.
- Reduce sodium intake to <2.4 g sodium or 6 g sodium chloride
- Stop smoking
- Reduce intake of dietary saturated fat and cholesterol

DRUG THERAPY
Initial drug therapy: use a diuretic or ß-Blocker if not contraindicated and no indications for another class of medications. ACE I, angiotensin-converting enzyme inhibitors; BPH, benign prostatic hyperplasia; CA, calcium antagonists; CS, cardioselective; DHP, dihydropyridine; ISA, intrinsic sympathomimetic activity; LA, long acting
Compelling Indications for certain clinical conditions:
 Diabetes mellitus- type I with proteinuria- ACE I
 Heart failure- ACE I, diuretics
 Isolated systolic hypertension (older patients)- diuretics (preferred), CA (LA DHP)
 Myocardial infarction- ß-Blocker (non-ISA), ACE I (with systolic dysfunction)
Possible favorable effects on Comorbid Conditions:
 Angina- ß-Blockers, CA; Atrial tachycardia or fibrillation- ß-Blockers, CA (non-DHP); BPH- α-Blockers; Diabetes Mellitus 1&2 with proteinuria- ACE I, CA; Diabetes Mellitus 2- diuretics; Dyslipidemia- α-Blockers; Essential tremors- ß-Blockers (non-CS); Heart failure- Carvedilol, losartan; Hyperthyroidism- ß-Blockers; Migraine- ß-Blockers (non-CS), CA (non-DHP); Myocardial Infarction- diltiazem, verapamil; Osteoporosis-thiazides; preoperative hypertension- ß-Blockers, Renal insufficiency (use caution in renovascular HTN)- ACE Inhibitors

HYPERTENSIVE CRISIS BP >200/120, symptoms- chest pain, headache, SOB, dizziness, blurred vision.
Goals to treatment: relief of symptoms, gradual improvement of BP to <160/110.

Hypertensive emergency- require immediate treatment to prevent or limit end organ damage, i.e.
cerebral edema (seizures, stupor, deficits, confusion), acute renal failure, LV failure, funduscopic (hemorrhage, exudates, A-V nicking, papilledema) or other neurological or vascular crisis (stroke). Requires hospitalization and parenteral antihypertensives (i.e. diazoxide, hydralazine, labetalol, nicardipine) in the ICU. Initial goal- reduce MAP no more than 25% within minutes to 2 hours, then 160/100 within 2-6 hours.

Hypertensive urgency- No ongoing end organ damage. Usually responds to oral agents with fast onset (loop diuretics, ß-Blockers, α2-agonists or CA): i.e. clonidine 0.2 mg initial dose then 0.1mg q hour up to 0.7mg total. Avoid use of sublingual fast acting nifedipine.

ACE INHIBITORS

It is recommended that diuretics be stopped 2-3 days prior to initial dose to avoid hypotension; diuretic therapy may be resumed if BP not controlled; hyperkalemia may result from concomitant use with K+ sparing diuretics or K+ supplements. Abbreviations for Approved Indication (AI) & Unlabeled uses (UL) as of NOV 1997 for HTN, CHF, LVD- left ventricular dysfunction, DN-diabetic nephropathy, RA- Raynaud's syndrome, HE-hypertensive emergency, AMI- acute myocardial infarction, increased survival if given within 24 hours

benazepril [Lotensin] (Tab 5, 15, 20, 40 mg) PO 10-40 mg QD. AI- HTN

captopril [Capoten] (Tab 12.5, 25, 50, 100 mg) PO 6.25-50 mg BID/TID, MAX 450 mg/24h, take 1hr before meals. AI- HTN, CHF, LVD, DN, AMI; UL- RA, HE

enalapril [Vasotec] (Tab 5, 10, 20 mg) PO 5-40 mg QD or +BID, MAX 40 mg/24h; IV (enalaprilat) 1.25 mg q 6h MAX 20 mg/24h. AI- HTN, CHF, LVD; UL- DN

fosinopril [Monopril] (Tab 10, 20 mg) PO 10-40 mg QD. AI- HTN, CHF

lisinopril [Prinivil, Zestril] (Tab 2.5, 5, 10, 20, 40 mg) PO 10-40 mg QD. AI- HTN, CHF, AMI

moexipril [Univasc] (Tab 7.5, 15 mg) PO 7.5-30 mg daily in 1 or 2 divided doses 1h prior to meal

perindopril [Aceon] (Tab 2, 4, 8 mg) PO 4-8mg QD. Max 16 mg/24h. AI- HTN

quinapril [Accupril] (Tab 5, 10, 20, 40 mg) PO 10-20 mg QD or 40-80 mg/D divided BID. AI- HTN, CHF

ramipril [Altace] (Tab 1.25, 2.5, 5, 10 mg) PO 2.5-20 mg QD or divided BID. AI- HTN, CHF

trandolapril [Mavik] (Tab 1, 2, 4 mg) PO 1mg QD initially; most patients require 2-4mg a day; Doses of 4 mg a day can be administered by twice daily dosing if once daily dosing provides inadequate control. AI- HTN

ANGIOTENSIN II RECEPTOR BLOCKERS

candesartan cilexetil [Atacand] (Tab 4, 8, 16, 32 mg) PO 2-32 mg QD, starting dose 16 mg QD; may be given once or twice daily. AI- HTN

eprosartan [Teveten] (Tab 600 mg) 400-800 mg once a day or may divide BID. AI- HTN ★

irbesartan [Avapro] (Tab 75, 150, 300 mg) 150-300 mg QD. AI- HTN

losartan potassium [Cozaar] (Tab 25, 50 mg) PO 25 mg QD initially, daily doses 25-100 mg can be administered once or twice daily. AI- HTN.

telmisartan [Micardis] (Tab 40, 80 mg) PO 20-80 mg QD. AI- HTN

valsartan[Diovan] (Cap 80, 160 mg) PO 80 mg QD initially, Maintenance 80-320 mg once daily. AI- HTN

ADRENERGIC AGONISTS (Central & Combinations)

clonidine [Catapres] (Tab 0.1, 0.2, 0.3 mg) PO 0.1-0.3 mg BID, MAX dose 2.4 mg/d

clonidine transdermal [Catapres-TTS] (Patch 0.1, 0.2, 0.3mg/D) 1 patch q week, MAX dose 0.6 mg/d

guanabenz [Wytensin] (Tab 4, 8 mg) PO 4-8 mg BID

guanfacine [Tenex] (Tab 1mg) PO 1 mg q HS

methyldopa [Aldomet] (Elx 250/5ml Tab 125, 250, 500 mg) PO 500 mg initially then 500-2000 mg divided BID/TID/QID; IV 250-500 mg q 6h, MAX 1000 mg/6h

ADRENERGIC BLOCKERS (Peripheral & Combinations)

<u>diazoxide</u> [Hyperstat] IV 1-3 mg/kg up to 150 mg q 5-15min

<u>doxazosin</u> [Cardura] (Tab 1, 2, 4, 8 mg) PO 1 mg QD initially, then up to 8 mg/D if needed.

<u>guanadrel</u> [Hylorel] (Tab 10, 25 mg) PO 5 mg BID initially, may increase to 20-75 mg/D +BID, MAX 400 mg/24h

<u>guanethidine</u> [Ismelin] (Tab 10, 25 mg) PO 10 mg QD initially, may increase to 25-50 mg QD

<u>phenoxybenzamine</u> [Dibenzyline] (Tab 10 mg) PO 10 mg BID, may increase to 20-40 mg BID/TID

<u>phentolamine</u> [Regitine] SC for extravasation for vasoconstrictors if given within 12h 5-10 mg in 10ml NS, IV for pheochromocytoma 5 mg increments

<u>prazosin</u> [Minipress] (Tab 1, 2, 5 mg) PO 1-5 mg BID/TID

<u>reserpine</u> [Serpasil] (Tab 0.1, 0.25, 1mg) PO 0.1-0.25 mg QD

<u>terazosin</u> [Hytrin] (Tab 1, 2, 5, 10 mg) PO 1 mg q HS, up to 10 mg q HS, MAX 20 mg/D

<u>trimethaphan</u> [Arfonad] IV 1-10 mg/min (500 mg in D₅W 100ml = 5 mg/ml)

ANTIANGINALS

<u>amyl nitrite</u> (Inhalant 0.3ml) 0.3 ml by inhalations Q 3-5 min prn

<u>isosorbide</u> [Ismotic] (Sol 45%) Initially 1.5 g/kg; then 1 to 3 g/kg 2 to 4 times a day ★

<u>isosorbide dinitrate</u> [Isordil, Sorbitrate] (Tab 5, 10, 20, 30, 40 mg; SR Tab 40 mg; SR Cap 40 mg; SL Tab 2.5, 5, 10 mg; Chew Tab 5, 10 mg)) PO 10-40 mg QID, SR 40-80 mg BID/TID; SL 1 q2-3h prn ★

<u>isosorbide mononitrate</u> [ISMO] (Tab 20 mg) PO 20 mg twice daily 7h apart

<u>isosorbide mononitrate</u> [Imdur ER, Isotrate ER] (Tab 30, 60, 120 mg) PO 30-120 mg qAM. (Max 240mg QD) ★

<u>nitroglycerin IV</u> [Tridil] 50 mg in D₅W or NS 250 ml (200 mcg/ml) 5-100 mcg/min titrate to relief or SE, use only in glass bottles and administration set provided.

<u>nitroglycerin SL</u> [Nitrostat] (Tab 0.15, 0.3, 0.4, 0.6 mg) SL 1 tab q 5 min prn angina, MAX 3 tabs/15 min

<u>nitroglycerin SL spray</u> [Nitrolingual] (0.4 mg/spray, 14.49 g bottle) 1 spray prn angina, MAX 3 sprays/15 min

<u>nitroglycerin, transmucosal</u> [Nitrogard] (Tab 1, 2, 3 mg) 1 tab between cheek & gum q3-5h while awake

<u>nitroglycerin ointment</u> [Nitro-Bid] (15 mg/inch) 0.5-2 inches upon rising and again 6 hs later.

<u>nitroglycerin patch</u> [Deponit 0.2, 0.4/Minitran 0.1, 0.2, 0.4, 0.6/Nitro-Dur 0.1, 0.2, 0.3, 0.4, 0.6,0.8/Nitrocine 0.6/ Nitrodisc 0.2, 0.3, 0.4/Transderm-Nitro 0.1, 0.2, 0.4, 0.6 mg/h] 1 QD for 12-14h then off for 10-12h

<u>pentaerythritol tetranitrate</u> [Peritrate] (Tab 10, 20, 40 mg, SR 30, 45 mg) PO 10-40 mg TID/QID, SR 1 tab q12h

ANTIARRHYTHMICS

<u>Classification</u> (C-conduction, P0D-Phase 0 depression, R-repolarization{↑ prolonged, ↓ shorten})

I	Sodium channel blockers	
	Ia	↓↓C, ↑R, ↓↓↓P0D: disopyramide, moricizine, procainamide, quinidine, tricyclics
	Ib	↓↓C, ↓R, ↓P0D: lidocaine, mexiletine, phenytoin, tocainide
	Ic	↓↓↓C, ↑R, ↓↓↓ P0D: encainide, flecainide, propafenone
II	Adrenergic blockers: acebutolol, esmolol, propranolol	
III	Prolonged repolarization: amiodarone, bretylium, sotalol	
IV	Calcium channel blockers: verapamil	
	Misc.: Digoxin, adenosine	

<u>adenosine</u> [Adenocard] (6 mg/2ml) IV initial dose 6 mg over 1-2 sec, then 12 mg within 1-2 min if needed, 12 mg may be repeated once if needed

<u>amiodarone</u> [Cordarone] (Tab 200 mg) a uniform dosing schedule has not been established, should only be administered by physicians who are experienced in amiodarone properties, close monitoring is essential due to serious potential SE. usual PO loading 800-1600 mg/d for 1-3 wk, maintenance 400 mg/d

<u>atropine</u> 0.4-1.0 mg IVP q1-2h

<u>bretylium</u> IV Load 5-10 mg/kg, drip 1-2 mg/min

<u>digitoxin</u> [Crystodigin] (Tab 0.05, 0.1, 0.15, 0.2 mg) PO Load 0.6 mg initially, followed by 0.4 mg 4-6h later, then 0.2 mg 4-6h later, then maintenance dose 0.05-0.3 mg QD

<u>digoxin</u> [Lanoxin/Lanoxicaps] (Elx 0.05 mg/ml Tab 0.125, 0.25, 0.5 mg /Caps 0.05, 0.1, 0.2 mg) PO 0.125-0.25 mg QD, IV loading 0.25 mg q6h up to 1 mg, (IV digitalizing dose is ≈ 20% less than oral dose. Lanoxicaps have increased bioavailability i.e. 0.1mg ≈ 0.125 mg standard tablet)

<u>digoxin Immune Fab</u> [Digibind] (40 mg/vial) IV 2-20 vials, 1 vial will bind 0.6mg of digoxin

<u>disopyramide</u> [Norpace/Norpace CR] (Tab 100,150/CR 100,150mg) PO 100-150 mg q6h; CR 200-300 mg q12h

<u>encainide</u> [Enkaid] (Tab 25, 35, 50 mg) PO 25 mg q 8h

<u>flecainide</u> [Tambocor] (Tab 50, 100, 150 mg) PO 50-150 mg q12h, MAX 400 mg/d

<u>ibutilide fumarate</u> [Corvert] (0.1mg/ml, 10 ml vials) IV over 10 min; initial dose (> 60 kg) 1 mg, (< 60 kg) 0.01mg/kg. Repeat dose if atrial fib/flutter continues. Stop immediately if arrhythmia terminates, Ventricular tachycardia occurs or prolongation of QT

<u>isoproterenol</u> : 1 mg in 500ml D₅W (2 µg/ml). Low dose is 2-10 µg/min. titrated to heart rate & rhythm response.

<u>lidocaine</u>: IV Load 1mg/kg, MAX 3 mg/kg; drip 1-4 mg/min, add 2 g in 250cc D5W (8 mg/ml) for drip.

<u>magnesium</u>: Dilute 1-2 g in 100 ml D₅W & give over 1-2 min in VF/VT. In pt. with documented Mg deficiency, load with 1-2 g in 50-100 ml D₅W give over 5-60 min & follow with infusion of 0.5-1 g/hr up to 24h.

mexiletine [Mexitil] (Tab 150, 200, 250 mg) PO 200-300 mg q8h, MAX 1200 mg/d
moricizine [Ethmozine] (Tab 200, 250, 300 mg) PO 150-300 mg TID
procainamide [Pronestyl] (Tab 250, 375, 500, Cap 250, 375, 500 mg, SR 250, 500, 750, 1000 mg) PO 50 mg/kg/24h divided q3-6h, SR q6h; IV see ACLS drugs above
propafenone [Rythmol] (Tab 150, 300 mg) PO 150-300 mg q8h, MAX 900 mg/d
quinidine gluconate [Quinaglute] (Tab 324 mg) PO 1 tab BID/TID
quinidine sulfate (Tab 200, 300 mg) PO 200-300 mg TID/QID
quinidine sulfate SR [Quinidex] (Tab 300 mg) PO 300-600 mg Q8-12h
tocainide [Tonocard] (Tab 400, 600 mg) PO 400-600 mg q 8h

HYPERLIPIDEMIA

CHD RISK FACTORS (RF): High risk if two or more POSITIVE risk factors are present
<u>POSITIVE RISK FACTORS:</u>
AGE: Male ≥45 y; Female ≥55 y or premature menopause without estrogen replacement
FAMILY HX: premature CHD- father or 1° ♂ relative with MI or sudden cardiac death before 55 years old, or mother or 1° ♀ relative <65 years of age
TOBACCO: current smoking
HYPERTENSION: 140/90 mmHg on several occasions or on antihypertensive medication.
DIABETES MELLITUS
LOW HDL CHOLESTEROL: <35 mg/dl
<u>NEGATIVE RISK FACTOR:</u> (if present may subtract one positive risk factor)
HIGH HDL CHOLESTEROL: ≥60 mg/dl

CLASSIFICATION OF CHOLESTEROL LEVELS

TOTAL CHOLESTEROL		HDL CHOLESTEROL	
Desirable	<200 mg/dL	Low	<35 mg/dL
Borderline-High	200-239 mg/dL		
High	≥ 240 mg/dL		

CURRENT TREATMENT RECOMMENDATIONS FOR HIGH CHOLESTEROL*
<u>PRIMARY PREVENTION*</u>

Total Cholesterol (mg/dL)..	HDL (mg/dL)	Treatment
<200	≥35	Repeat Total & HDL within 5 y. Provide education.
	<35	Do lipoprotein analysis, based on LDL- see below
200-239	≥35	If <2 RF, provide info on modification, recheck 1-2 y
	<35	or ≥2 RF, lipoprotein analysis, based on LDL- see below
>240		Do lipoprotein analysis, based on LDL- see below

LDL Cholesterol (mg/dL)	Risk Factors	
<130		Repeat Total & HDL within 5 y. Provide education.
130-159	<2	Provide info on step 1 diet & exercise, recheck annually
	≥2	Initiate dietary therapy, see SECONDARY PREVENTION
≥160		Initiate dietary therapy, see SECONDARY PREVENTION

<u>SECONDARY PREVENTION</u> * based on LDL (mg/dL) **Calculated LDL**= total cholesterol - HDL - TG/5
≤ 100 .... Repeat analysis annually. Diet & physical activity
>100 .... Initiate therapy

<u>DIETARY THERAPY*</u>	LDL Initiation Level	LDL goal
<2 RF	≥160	<160 mg/dL
≥ 2 RF	≥130	<130
Known CHD		≤100

<u>CONSIDER DRUG THERAPY*</u>	LDL Level	LDL goal
<2 RF	≥190†	<160 mg/dL
≥2 RF	≥160	<130
Known CHD	>130‡	≤100

† drug therapy in high risk patients (diabetes) should be initiated; otherwise delay drug therapy and initiate dietary therapy in male <35yrs and premenopausal female. ‡ Clinical judgment in deciding to initiate drug therapy. * Data from 2nd Report of the Expert Panel on Detection, Evaluation, and Treatment of High Blood Cholesterol; NIH Sept 1993

ANTILIPIDS (BAS-bile acid sequestrants, HMG-HMG-CoA reductase inhibitors, CAT-increased catabolism)
atorvastatin [Lipitor] HMG (Tabs 10, 20, 40 mg) 10-80 mg/D with or without food
cerivastatin [Baycol] HMG (Tab 0.2, 0.3 mg) 0.3 mg tab q PM; use 0.2 mg with CrCl ≤60 ml/min.
cholestyramine [Cholybar, Questran] BAS (Bar or powder 4g) PO 4 gm 1-6/D
clofibrate [Atromid-S] (Tab 500 mg) PO 1 tab QID

colestipol [Colestid] BAS (Tab 5g) PO 1-2 tabs TID/QID
dextrothyroxine [Choloxin] CAT (Tab 1, 2, 4, 6mg) PO 1-2 mg QD, then ↑ q month as needed, MAX 8 mg/D
fenofibrate [Tricor] (Caps 67 mg) initial dose 67 mg/D given with meal. MAX dose 201mg/D ★
fenofibrate [Lipidil] (Cap 100 mg) PO 100 mg QD
fluvastatin [Lescol] HMG (Tab 20, 40 mg) PO 20-40 mg QD in the evening without regard to meals
gemfibrozil [Lopid] (Tab 300, 600 mg) PO 600 mg BID 30min before morning & evening meals
niacin [Niacor] (Tab 500 mg) PO 1-2 gm TID with or after meals, MAX 8 g/D
niacin [Niaspan] [ext-rel Tab 375, 500, 750, 1000 mg) *Starter pack* 375 mg QD X 1 wk, then 500 mg QD 2ⁿᵈ wk,
    then 750 mg 3ʳᵈ wk, then 1 g QD for 4ᵗʰ-7ᵗʰ wk May ↑ 500 mg every 4 wks to response. Max 2 g/D ★
lovastatin [Mevacor] HMG (Tab 10, 20, 40 mg) PO 20-40 mg qd with evening meal, MAX 80 mg/D. SE: ↑
    serum transaminase, monitor LFT q 6wks for 1st year; then q 8wks for 1st year; then q 6m
probucol [Lorelco] CAT (Tab 250, 500 mg) PO 500 mg BID with morning & evening meal
pravastatin [Pravachol] HMG (Tab 10, 20 mg) PO 10-40 mg q HS
simvastatin [Zocor] HMG (Tab 5, 10, 20, 40, 80★ mg) PO 5-80 mg QD in the evening

CLASSIFICATION OF HYPERLIPIDEMIA

Type	I	IIa	IIb	III	IV	V
Cholesterol	=↑	↑	↑	=↑	=↑	=↑
Triglycerides	↑	=	↑	=↑	↑	↑
Chylomicrons	↑	=	=	=	=	↑
VLDL	=↑	=↓	=	=	=	=
LDL	↓	↑	↑	↑	=↓	↓
HDL	↓	=	=	=	↓	↓
Treatment	D	D, CH, CO, DE, NA, PR, ST	D, CH, CO, CL, GE, NA, PR, ST	D, CL, NA	D, CL, GE, NA	D, CL, GE, NA

=-normal/no change, ↑-increased, ↓-decreased, D-diet, CH-cholestyramine, CL-clofibrate,
CO-colestipol, DE-dextrothyroxine, NA-nicotinic acid, PR-probucol, ST-statins, GE-gemfibrozil

ANTIHYPERLIPIDEMIC EFFECTS

DRUG	CH	CL	CO	DE	GE	ST	NA	PR
Cholesterol	↓	↓	↓	↓	↓	↓	↓	↓
Triglycerides	=↑	↓	=↑	=	↓	↓	↓	=
VLDL	=↑	↓	↑	=	↓	↓	↓	↑↓
LDL	↓	=↓	↓	↓	=↓	↓	↓	↓
HDL	=↑	=↑	=↑	↑	↑	↑	↑	↓

β ADRENERGIC BLOCKERS

acebutolol [Sectral] (Tab 200, 400 mg) β1; PO 200 mg BID or 400 mg QD
atenolol [Tenormin] (Tab 25, 50, 100 mg) β1; PO 25-100 mg QD, IV 5 mg over 5min may repeat in 10min
betaxolol [Kerlone] (Tab 10, 20 mg) β1; PO 10-20 mg QD
bisoprolol fumarate [Zebeta] (Tab 5, 10 mg) β1; PO 2.5-20 mg QD
carteolol [Cartrol] (Tab 2.5, 5 mg) β1, β2; PO 2.5-5 mg QD
carvedilol [Coreg] (Tab 3.125, 6.25, 12.5, 25 mg) *HTN initially* 6.25 mg BID, ↑ at 1-2 week intervals to 12.5 mg
    BID, (MAX 25 mg BID); *CHF initially* 3.125 mg BID, ↑ at 2 week intervals as tolerated, (MAX <85kg 25 mg
    BID, >85kg 50 mg BID)
esmolol [Brevibloc] β1, β2; IV 50-200 mcg/kg/min (5g in 500ml NS/D₅/D₅NS/D₅½NS) MAX 300mcg/kg/min
labetalol [Normodyne,Trandate](Tab100,200,300mg)α1,β1,β2,PO100-400mg BID,IV 20mg q10min Max 300mg
metoprolol [Lopressor] (Tab 50, 100 mg) β1; PO 50-200 mg BID MAX 450 mg/D, IV 5 mg up to 15 mg.
metoprolol [Toprol XL] (Tab 50, 100, 200mg) PO 50-400 mg QD ★
nadolol [Corgard] (Tab 20, 40, 80, 120, 160 mg) β1, β2; PO 40-160 mg QD
penbutolol [Levatol] (Tab 20 mg) β1, β2; PO 20-40 mg QD
pindolol [Visken] (Tab 5, 10 mg) 1, 2; PO 5-20 mg BID, MAX 60 mg/D
propranolol [Inderal] (Tab 10, 20, 40, 60, 80, 90 SR 60, 80, 120, 160 mg; IV 1 mg/ml) α1, β1, β2; PO 40-60 mg
    BID/TID/QID, SR 80- 120 mg q D, IV 1-3 mg (push Max 1 ml/min) may repeat in 2 min then in 4h
sotalol [Betapace] (Tab 80, 160, 240 mg) β1, β2; PO 80-160 mg BID
timolol [Blocadren] (Tab 5, 10, 20 mg) β1, β2; PO 10-20 mg BID

CALCIUM CHANNEL BLOCKERS

<u>amlodipine</u> [Norvasc] (Tab 2.5, 5, 10 mg) PO 5-10 mg QD, MAX 10 mg/D

<u>bepridil</u> [Vascor] (Tab 200, 300, 400 mg) PO 200-400 mg QD, MAX 400 mg/D

<u>diltiazem</u> [Cardizem] (CD Cap 120, 180, 240, 300 mg; Injectable 25 mg/5ml, 50 mg/10ml; Lyo-Ject 25 mg syringe; Monovial 100 mg/vial for continuous infusion) PO CD 120-480 mg QD; IV or Lyo-Ject 20 mg (0.25 mg/kg) over 2 min., then 25 mg (0.35 mg/kg) if needed in 15 min., then 5-15 mg/h IV infusion for up to 24 hrs.

<u>diltiazem</u> [Dilacor XR] (Tab 120, 180, 240 mg) 180-480 mg once a day.

<u>diltiazem</u> [Tiazac] (Tab 120, 180, 240, 300, 360, 420 mg) PO 120-540 mg once a day ★

<u>felodipine</u> [Plendil] (Tab 2.5, 5, 10 mg) PO 2.5-10 mg QD

<u>isradipine</u> [DynaCirc] (Tab 2.5, 5 mg) PO 2.5-5 mg BID, MAX 20 mg/D

<u>mibefradil</u> [Posicor] withdrawn from market ★

<u>nicardipine</u> [Cardene] (Tab 20, SR 30 30, 45, 60 mg) PO 20-40 mg TID, SR 30 mg BID, IV 5-15 mg/h

<u>nifedipine</u> [Adalat, Procardia] (Tab 10, 20; CC or XL 30, 60, 90 mg) PO 10-30 mg TID, MAX 180 mg/D; CC or XL 30-60 mg QD, MAX 120 mg/D

<u>nimodipine</u> [Nimotop] (Tab 30 mg) Subarachnoid hemorrhage PO 60 mg q 4h for 21 days

<u>nisoldipine</u> [Sular] (Tab 10, 20, 30, 40 mg) 10-40 mg PO QD. HTN

<u>verapamil</u> [Calan, Isoptin] (Tab 40, 80, 120; SR 120, 180, 240 mg; 5 mg/ml) PO 80-120 mg TID, SR 120-240 mg QD, SIVP 0.1-0.3 mg/kg up to 5-20 mg.

<u>verapamil</u> [Covera- HS] (Tab 180, 240 mg) PO 180-540 mg at HS

DIURETICS (CAI- carbonic anhydrase inhibitor, KS- K+ sparing, TH- thiazide)

<u>acetazolamide</u> [Diamox] CAI (Tab 125, 250, 500 mg) PO/IV 250-375 mg QOD

<u>Aldactazide</u> [HCTZ/spironolactone] TH/KS (25/25, 50/50) PO 1-4 tabs QD

<u>amiloride</u> [Midamor] KS (Tab 5 mg) PO 5-15 mg QD

<u>bendroflumethiazide</u> [Naturetin] (Tab 5, 10 mg) PO 5-20 mg QD

<u>benzthiazide</u> [Exna] (Tab 50 mg) PO 25-50 mg BID, MAX 200 mg/D

<u>bumetanide</u> [Bumex] Loop (Tab 0.5, 1, 2 mg) PO/IM/IV 0.5-2 mg QD

<u>chlorothiazide</u> [Diuril] TH (Tab 250, 500 Susp 250 mg/5ml) PO/IV 50-1000 mg QD/BID

<u>chlorthalidone</u> [Hygroton] TH (Tab 25, 50, 100 mg) PO 25-100 mg QD

<u>dichlorphenamide</u> [Daranide] CAI (Tab 50 mg) PO 100 mg BID

<u>Dyazide</u> [HCTZ/triamterene] TH/KS (Tab 25/25 mg) PO 1-2 tabs QD/BID

<u>ethacrynic acid</u> [Edecrin] Loop (Tab 25, 50 mg) IV 0.5-1.0 mg/kg up to 50 mg; PO 25-100 mg QD/BID

<u>furosemide</u> [Lasix] Loop (Tab 20, 40, 80 mg) PO 20-80 mg QD/BID; IV 1 mg/kg up to 20-40 mg

<u>hydrochlorothiazide</u> [Esidrix] TH (Tab 25, 50, 100 mg) PO 25-100 mg QD/BID

<u>hydroflumethiazide</u> [Diucardin] TH (Tab 50 mg) PO 50 mg QD/BID, MAX 200 mg/24h

<u>indapamide</u> [Lozol] TH (Tab 1.25, 2.5 mg) PO 2.5-5 mg QD, MAX 5 mg/24h

<u>mannitol</u> [Osmitrol] (5%, 10%, 15%, & 20% for IV infusion) 20-200 g/24h; maintain 30-50ml/hr urine output. *Test Dose*: 0.2 g/kg infused over 3-5 min. *Increased intracranial pressure*: 1.5-2 g/kg of 15-20% solution over 30-60 min, monitor serum osmolality.

<u>Maxzide</u> [HCTZ/triamterene] TH/KS (Tab 25/37.5, 50/75 mg) PO 1-2 25/37.5 tabs or 1 50/75 mg QD

<u>methazolamide</u> [Neptazane] CAI (Tab 50 mg) PO 50-100 mg BID/TID glaucoma

<u>methyclothiazide</u> [Aquatensen, Enduron] TH (Tab 2.5, 5 mg) PO 2.5-10 mg QD

<u>metolazone</u> [Zaroxolyn] TH (Tab 2.5, 5, 10 mg) PO 2.5-5 mg QD

<u>Moduretic</u> [HCTZ/amiloride] TH/KS (Tab 50/5 mg) PO 1-2 tabs QD with meals

<u>polythiazide</u> [Renese] TH (Tab 1, 2, 4 mg) PO 1-4 mg QD

<u>quinethazone</u> [Hydromox] (Tab 50 mg) PO 50-100 mg QD

<u>spironolactone</u> [Aldactone] KS (Tab 25, 50, 100 mg) PO 25-100 mg QD/BID

<u>torsemide</u> [Demadex] loop(Tab 5, 10, 20, 100 mg) PO/IV 5-20 mg QD MAX 200 mg/24h,IV & PO ≈ equivalent

<u>triamterene</u> [Dyrenium] KS (Tab 50, 100 mg) PO 100 mg BID, MAX 300 mg/d

<u>trichlormethiazide</u> [Naqua] TH (Tab 2, 4 mg) PO 2-4 mg QD

COMBINATION ANTIHYPERTENSIVES

<u>Aldoclor</u> [chlorothiazide/methyldopa] (Tab 150/250, 250/250 mg) PO 1 tabs BID/QID

<u>Aldoril</u> [HCTZ/methyldopa] (Tab 15/250, 25/250 30/500, 50/500 mg) PO 1 tab TID

<u>Apresazide</u> [HCTZ/hydralazine] (Tab 25/25, 50/50, 100/100 mg) PO 1 tab BID

<u>Avalide</u> [irbesartan /HCTZ] (Tab 150mg/12.5mg, 300mg/12.5mg) 1 tab QD (Max 150/12.5 tabs daily)★

<u>Combipres</u> [clonidine/chlorthalidone] (Tab 0.1mg/15mg, 0.2mg/15mg, 0.3mg/15mg) 1 tab QD-BID★

<u>Capozide</u> [captopril/HCTZ] (Tab 25/15, 25/25, 50/15, 50/25 mg) PO 1 tab BID

<u>Corzide</u> [nadolol/bendroflumethiazide] (Tab 40/5, 80mg/5mg) 40-80 mg QD. Up to 240-320 mg QD ★

<u>Diovan HCT</u> [HCTZ] (Tab 80mg/12.5mg, 160mg/12.5mg) 1 tab QD; (Max two 80mg/12.5mg tabs QD)★

<u>Esimil</u> [guanethidine/HCTZ] (Tab 10/25 mg) PO 1-2 tab QD

<u>Hyzaar</u> 50-12.5 or 100-25 [losartan/HCTZ] (Tab 50mg/12.5mg, 100mg/25mg) One 50mg/12.5mg tab QD, may titrate after 2-3 weeks to 100mg/25mg QD ★

<u>Inderide</u> [propranolol/HCTZ] (Tab 40/25, 80/25 mg) PO 1-2 tabs QD/BID
<u>Inderide LA</u> [propranolol/HCTZ] (Tab 80/50, 120/50, 160/50 mg) PO 1 tab QD
<u>Lexxel</u> [enalapril 5 mg/felodipine 5 mg] 1 tab QD. HTN
<u>Lotrel</u> [amlodipine/benazepril] (Cap 2.5/10, 5/10, 5/20 mg) PO 1 Cap QD
<u>metyrosine</u> [Demser] (Tab 250 mg) PO 250-1000 mg QID, MAX 4 gm/D
<u>Minizide</u> [prazosin/polythiazide] (Tab 1/0.5, 2/0.5, 5/0.5 mg) PO 1 tab BID
<u>Normozide</u> [labetalol/HCTZ] (Tab 100/25, 200/25, 300/25 mg) PO 1 tab BID
<u>Prinzide</u> [lisinopril/HCTZ] (Tab 20/25, 20/12.5 mg) PO 1-2 tabs QD
<u>reserpine</u> [Serpasil] (Tab 0.1, 0.25, 1mg) PO 0.1-0.25 mg QD
<u>Teczem</u> [enalapril 5 mg + diltiazem 180 mg] (Ext Release Tab) Titrate individual components. *HTN*
<u>Tenoretic</u> [atenolol/chlorthalidone] (Tab 50/25, 100/25 mg) PO 1 tab QD
<u>Timolide</u> [timolol/HCTZ] (Tab 10/25 mg) PO 1 tab BID
<u>Trandate HCT</u> [labetalol/HCTZ] (Tab 100/25, 200/25, 300/25 mg) PO 1 tab BID
<u>Vaseretic</u> [enalapril/HCTZ] (Tab 10/25 mg) PO 1 tab QD
<u>Zestoretic</u> [lisinopril/HCTZ] (Tab 20/12.5, 20/25 mg) PO 1-2 tabs QD
<u>Ziac</u> [bisoprolol fumarate/HCTZ] (Tab 2.5/6.25, 5/6.25, 10/6.25 mg) PO 2.5-10 mg QD

CONTRAINDICATIONS TO THROMBOLYTIC THERAPY

ABSOLUTE	RELATIVE
· Active bleeding	· Potential hemorrhagic focus
· Suspected Aortic Dissection	a) diabetic proliferative retinopathy
· Acute pericarditis	b) GI or GU hemorrhage or stroke(*6 months*)
· Previous documented allergic reaction to or recent (4d-12mo) use of SK or APSAC (use tPA)	c) major surgery, organ biopsy, major trauma, puncture of non-compressible vessel, prolonged chest compressions, minor head trauma ($\leq$2-4 weeks)
· Previous cerebral hemorrhage, intracerebral vascular disease (aneurysm, AVM), cerebral neoplasm	d) diabetic proliferative retinopathy
	e) severe uncontrolled HTN (*SBP >200 or DBP >120*)
	· History of bleeding diathesis, Cancer, Hepatic dysfunction.
	· Pregnancy

4ᵗʰ Cons on Antithrombotic Therapy; *Chest* OCT 1995 S

THROMBOLYTICS/ANTICOAGULANTS/MISCELLANEOUS BLOOD MODIFIERS

<u>albumin</u> [Albuminar-5&25] (5, 25%) IV dose dependent on clinical condition
<u>alteplase</u> [Activase, TPA] *accelerated infusion*- 15 mg IV over 1-2min, then 50 mg (0.75 mg/kg if ≤67 kg)over 30 min, 35 mg (0.5 mg/kg if ≤67 kg) over next 60 min; 3 hour infusion- 60 mg infused over the 1ˢᵗ hour (6-10 mg bolus over the 1ˢᵗ 1-2 minutes, then 20 mg/h for the next 2 hours. Heparin 5,000u IVP then 1,000u/h if <85kg or 1,200u/h if >85kg. Acute ischemic stroke- 0.9 mg/kg (90 mg max) infused over 60 minutes with 10% of the dose given over the 1ˢᵗ minute. Pulmonary embolus- 100 mg infusion over 2 hours.
<u>anagrelide</u> [Agrylin] (Tab 0.5, 1mg) Start 0.5 mg PO QID or 1 mg BID, maintain for ≥1 week then adjust to lowest dose to maintain platelet count <600,000/ml (MAX 10 mg/day or 2.5 mg single dose)
<u>anistreplase</u> [APSAC, Eminase] IV 30 units over 2-5 min
<u>aprotinin</u> [Trasylol] protease inhibitor to reduce perioperative blood loss in patients undergoing CABG. IV 2 million KIU loading dose, 2 million KIU pump prime, and 500,000 KIU/h continuous infusion during operation.
<u>ardeparin sodium</u> [Normiflo] (Injection 5000, 10,000 anti-Xa U/0.5ml) 50 anti-Xa U/kg deep SC q 12h
<u>cilostazol</u> [Pletal] (Tab 50, 100 mg) 100 mg PO BID; consider 50 mg BID if taking along with inhibitors of CYP3A4 (e.g., ketoconazole, itraconazole, erythromycin, or diltiazem, or CYP2C19 inhibitors such as omeprazole.) *phosphodiesterase III inhibitor* for Intermittent claudication ★
<u>clopidogrel</u> [Plavix] (Tab 75 mg) One tab PO QD with or without food. *Irreversible inhibition* ★
<u>danaparoid</u> [Orgaran] (750 anti-Xa units/0.6ml) Hip replacement DVT prophylaxis SC 0.6ml BID
<u>dipyridamole</u> [Persantine] Tab 25, 50, 75 mg PO 75-100 mg QID
<u>dalteparin sodium</u> [Fragmin] (Sol 16, 32 mg/0.2ml) *DVT prophylaxis use* 2500-5000 IU QD; *Systemic anticoagulation use* 200IU/kg deep SC QD or 100 IU/kg deep SC BID
<u>dextran</u> Shock IV Dextran 40: 10 ml/kg rapidly; Dextran 70: 500-100ml at 20-40ml/min, MAX 20ml/kg first 24h
<u>enoxaparin</u> [Lovenox] (Pre-filled syringes 30mg/.3ml, 40mg/.4ml, 60mg/.6ml, 80mg/.8ml, 100mg/1ml) prevention of DVT following hip replacement SC 30 mg BID while inpatient and outpatient home use for up to 3 weeks following hip replacement surgery with SC 40 mg QD. Prevention of DVT in patients undergoing abdominal or knee surgery 40 mg SC QD. Prevention of ischemic complications of unstable angina and non-Q-wave MI
<u>eptifibatide</u> [Integrilin] (Inj 0.75 mg/ml, 2 mg/ml vials) *Acute coronary syndrome* 180 mcg/kg IV ASAP following Dx, follow with 2 mcg/kg/min IV drip until hospital discharge or initiation of CABG, up to 72 hours ★
<u>heparin</u> [Liquaemin] (1000, 5000, 10000, 20000 &40000u/ml) IV/SC; Low dose prophylaxis SC 5000u q8-12h
<u>hetastarch</u> [Hespan] (6g in 100ml NS) IV volume expansion 500-1000 ml, MAX 1500 ml/D

lepirudin [Refludan] (50 mg/vial) For anticoagulation in patients with heparin-induced thrombocytopenia and associated thromboembolic disease to prevent further thromboembolic complications. Initial bolus - 0.4 mg/kg body weight (up to 110 kg) IV (slowly, over 15-20 sec), followed by a continuous IV infusion of 0.15 mg/kg/hr for 2-10 days or longer if clinically indicated

pentoxifylline [Trental] (Tab 400 mg) PO 400 mg TID

protamine sulfate (10 mg/ml) SIVP(over 10min) 1mg neutralizes 90-115 units of heparin, MAX 50 mg/Dose. *Rapid injection may result in hypotension &/or anaphylactoid reaction.*

ticlopidine [Ticlid] (Tab 250 mg) PO 250 mg BID with food

tirofiban [Aggrastat] glucoprotein IIb/IIIa receptor antagonist for use with heparin for treatment of acute coronary syndrome; IV at an initial rate of 0.4 mcg/kg/min for 30 minutes and then 0.1 mcg/kg/min

streptokinase [Streptase] IV 1.5 million units over 60 min

warfarin [Coumadin] (Tab 1, 2, 2.5, 4, 5, 7.5, 10 mg) PO 10 mg/D for 2-4 days then maintenance of 2-10 mg daily based on INR. Warfarin reduces the synthesis of Vit. K dependent clotting Factors (II, VII [1st to ↓], IX, X).

VASODILATORS

diazoxide [Hyperstat] IV 1-3 mg/kg, max 150 mg/dose, may be repeated at 5-15 min intervals

hydralazine [Apresoline] (Tab 10, 25, 50, 100 mg) PO 10-50 mg QID, IM/IV 20-40 mg q 4-6h

minoxidil [Loniten] (Tab 2.5, 10 mg) PO 5-40 mg QD, MAX 100 mg/D

Nitroglycerin: 50 or 100 mg in 250cc D₅W or NS, start at 10-20 mcg/min, increase by 5-10 mcg/min q 5-10 min. Low doses = mainly venodilation; high doses = arteriolar dilation also.

nitroprusside sodium [Nipride] IV 0.5-10 mcg/kg/min (50 [or 100 mg] in D₅W 250 ml = 250 mcg/ml [500]) monitor thiocyanate levels at ↑ doses (wrap solution & tubing in opaque material).

trimethaphan camsylate [Arfonad] (50 mg/ml) Start at 3-4 mg/min IV, titrate to effect

VASOPRESSORS/INOTROPIC/CHRONOTROPIC AGENTS

amrinone lactate [Inocor] 0.75mcg/kg IV slow push over 2-3min, Maintenance 5-10mcg/kg/min (MAX 10 mg/kg/d)

dobutamine [Dobutrex] Usual dose is 2-20 mcg/kg/min (1000 mg in 250cc D₅W or NS) Heart rate increases, especially at higher doses - this may exacerbate myocardial ischemia.

dopamine Add 400 mg to 250ml D₅W (1600 mcg/ml); IV 2-50 mcg/kg/min, doses of 2-5 mcg/kg/min are predominately dopaminergic & β- agonist; doses >10 mcg/kg/min are α-agonist.

ephedrine SC/IM 25-50 mg, slow IV 10-25 mg, MAX 150 mg/D

epinephrine As vasopressor dose, 1mg in 500 ml D₅W or NS & start with 1mcg/min continuous drip titrated to response. During cardiac arrest, epi may be given as a continuous infusion - add 30 mg epi to 250ml D₅W or NS & run at 100 ml/hr (comparable to the standard 1 mg dosing).Alternate Epi dosing regimens: Intermediate: epi 2-5 mg q 3-5 min; Escalating: epi 1mg- 3mg- 5 mg 3 min apart; High: epi 0.1 mg/kg q 3-5 min

isoproterenol [Isuprel] IV bolus initial 0.02-0.06 mg, subsequent bolus 0.01-0.2 mg, drip 5 mcg/min

metaraminol [Aramine] IV 15-100 mg in 250-100 ml NS or D5 adjust rate to desired blood pressure

milrinone lactate [Primacor] loading 50 mcg/kg IV over 10 min, maintenance 0.375-0.75 mcg/kg/min, MAX 1.13 mg/kg/d

norepinephrine [Levophed] Add 4mg norepinephrine (16 mcg/ml) or 8mg norepinephrine bitartrate (32 mcg/ml) to 250ml D₅W with or without saline; begin with 0.5-1 mcg/min IV drip & titrate, average 2-4 mcg/min.

phenylephrine [Neo-Synephrine] SC/IM 2-5mg; IV 0.2mg, IV drip(10mg in 250ml NS or D5) start 40-180mcg/min

Cardiology Notes:

EQUATIONS [Normal Values]

$$\text{Mean Arterial Pressure} = \frac{SBP + 2(DBP)}{3} \quad [75 - 110\,mmHg]$$

$$\text{Stroke Volume} = \frac{(1000\,ml/l)\,(C.O.)}{\text{Heart Rate}} \quad [60 - 100\,ml/beat]$$

$$\text{Ejection Fraction} = \frac{\text{Stroke Volume (SV)}}{\text{End Diastolic Volume (EDV)}} \quad [56 - 78\%]$$

$$\text{Stroke Volume Index} = \frac{\text{Stroke Volume}}{\text{Body Surface Area (BSA)}} \quad [30 - 60\,ml/beat/m^2]$$

$$\text{Cardiac Index} = \frac{\text{Cardiac Output}}{\text{Body Surface Area}} \quad [2.5 - 4.0\,l/beat/m^2]$$

$$\text{Cardiac Output} = \text{Stroke Volume} \times \text{Heart Rate} \quad [5 - 8\,l/min]$$

$$\text{Cardiac Output Estimate} = \frac{O_2\,\text{uptake} \times BSA}{\Delta(A-V)\%O_2\,Sat \times 10} \quad [5 - 8\,l/min]$$

Use O_2 Uptake estimate ($\dot{V}O_2$): old = 110; average = 125; burn, septic = 140 cc/m²/min

$\dot{V}O_2 = \text{cardiac index} \times \Delta(A-V)\%O_2\,Sat \times 10 \quad [110 - 160\,ml/min/m^2]$

$\Delta(A-V)\%O_2\,Sat = 1.38Hgb \times (\text{arterial}\,\%O_2\,Sat - \text{mixed venous}\,\%O_2\,Sat) \quad [4 - 6\,ml/dl]$

O_2 Extraction Ratio = $\dot{V}O_2/\dot{D}O_2 \quad [22 - 32\%]$

$\dot{D}O_2 = \text{cardiac index} \times 1.38Hgb \times \text{arterial}\,\%O_2\,Sat \times 10 \quad [500 - 600\,ml/min/m^2]$

$$\text{Systemic Vascular Resist. (SVR)} = \frac{MAP - RAm}{\text{Cardiac Output}} \times 80 \quad [900 - 1400\,dynes \times sec \times cm^{-5}]$$

$$\text{SVR Index} = \frac{MAP - RAm}{\text{Cardiac Index}} \times 80 \quad [900 - 1400\,dynes \times sec \times cm^{-5} \times m^2]$$

$$\text{Pulmonary vascular resistance} = \frac{PAPm - PCWPm}{\text{Cardiac Output}} \times 80 \quad [100 - 250\,dynes \times sec \times cm^{-5}]$$

$$\text{PVR Index} = \frac{PAPm - PCWPm}{\text{Cardiac Index}} \times 80 \quad [200 - 450\,dynes \times sec \times cm^{-5} \times m^2]$$

$$\text{Double Product} = \frac{\text{Heart Rate} \times \text{Systolic Blood Pressure}}{100} \quad [60 - 140]$$

TYPICAL HEMODYNAMIC MEASUREMENTS DURING VARIOUS SHOCK STATES

DIAGNOSIS	BP	HR	CO	SV	PCWP	PAP	CVP
Normal	120/80	80	6	70	10	25/10	5
Septic, early	↓	↑	↑	↑	↓	=	↓
Late	↓	↑↓	N	↑↓	↑	N	N
Terminal	↓	↓↓	↓	↑	↑	↑	↑
Cardiogenic (LV infarct)	↓↓	↑	↓	↓↓	↑↑	↑/↑	↑
Tamponade	↓↓	↑	↓	↓↓	↑	↑/↑	↑↑
Pulmonary HTN	↓↓	↑	↓	↓↓	=	↑↑/↑↑	↑
RV infarction	↓↓	↑	↓	↓↓	=	↑/↓	↑
Hypovolemic	↓↓	↑	↓	↓↓	↓	↓↓↓	↓
Neurogenic	↓↓↓	=	↓	↓	↓	↓↓↓↓	↓
Anaphylactic	↓↓	↑	↓	↓	↓	↓↓↓↓	↓
Adrenal insufficiency	↓↓	↑	↓	↓	↓	↓↓↓↓	↓

ACUTE RESPIRATORY DISTRESS SYNDROME (ARDS)

Characteristics

Predisposing insult resulting in noncardiogenic pulmonary capillary leakage. (See DDX) Ensuing alveolar and interstitial edema develops. Followed by rapidly progressive hypoxemia, decreased lung compliance and diffused pulmonary infiltrates. PCWP remains normal, distinguishing ARDS from cardiogenic pulmonary edema. Mortality 50-70%.

DDX

Pulmonary	Non pulmonary
Diffuse infection	Sepsis
Toxin inhalation	Shock
Trauma	Septic
Aspiration	Hypovolemic
Airway contusion	Cardiogenic
Near-drowning	Cardiopulmonary bypass
	Hypertransfusion
	Drugs
	Pancreatitis
	Trauma- Massive non-thoracic
	Immunologic disorders
	Hematologic disorders
	Uremia
	CNS disease

Treatment

- Maintain Pa_{O2} >60 mmHg (O_2 saturation of >90%) with the lowest possible Fl_{O2},
- Mechanical ventilatory support
  Decrease Fl_{O2} from 100% to <60% as tolerated
  Add PEEP if needed to keep Fl_{O2} <60% and Pa_{O2} >60 mmHg
      Start at 5 cmH$_2$O, increase by 3-5 cmH$_2$O if needed to a maximum of 15 cmH$_2$O
  Lowest tidal volume 6-10 mL/kg
  Adjust minute volume to maintain pH above 7.25
- Treat underlying cause,
- Hemodynamic and nutritional support
- Possible complications: Oxygen toxicity, barotrauma from mechanical ventilation, DIC, LV failure, secondary bacterial infection, multisystem organ failure.

[1]*Harrison's Principles of Internal Medicine*, 14th ed, Braunwald E (ed). New York, McGraw-Hill, 1998, pp 1483-1486. [1]*Cecil's Textbook of Internal Medicine*, 20th ed, Wyngaarden JB, Smith LH, and Bennett K (eds). Philadelphia, Saunders, 1997

PULMONARY EMBOLISM

Characteristics

90% arise from DVT of the legs and pelvis.

Predisposing factors: Trauma, surgery, cancer, pregnancy, obesity, CHF, oral contraceptives, immobility, MI, previous DVT, nephrotic syndrome, other hypercoagulable states/conditions.

Prophylactic therapy: low dose heparin 5,000 units SC q8-12 hours or low molecular weight heparin (enoxaparin 30mg SC BID), Intermittent Pneumatic Compression Device

Presenting Symptoms: chest pain, SOB, cough, hemoptysis

Signs: tachycardia, tachypnea, cardiogenic shock

CXR- usually normal. May show effusion, atelectasis, infiltrate ("wedge sign", elevated hemidiaphragm, cut off sign (hyperlucency of lung parenchyma)

Diagnosis

- V/Q scan- Essentially rules out PE if normal. High probability- treat for PE. Indeterminate- get angiography. Negative adequate angiogram rules out PE. Positive angiogram- confirms PE. Treatment: heparin 5,000-10,000u (100u/kg)IV bolus followed by 1,000-1,500 u/h (20u/kg/h) IV drip; Monitor PTT q6h, adjust heparin to obtain and maintain PTT of 50-80 sec or or low molecular weight heparin (enoxaparin 1 mg/kg SC q12° or 1.5 mg/kg qD). Start warfarin on day 2 if heparin is therapeutic. Overlap heparin and warfarin for at least 4 days. May d/c heparin when INR is 2.0-3.0 for 2 consecutive days. Consider Thrombolytics for massive PE.

HEMODYNAMIC TRENDS OF COMMON CARDIAC DRUGS

DRUG	BP	HR	CO	SV	SVR	PCWP
DOPAMINE (<6 µg/kg/min)	0 to ↓	↑	↑↑	↑	0 to ↓	=
(>6µg/kg/min)	↑↑		↑↓			
DOBUTAMINE	0 to ↑	0 to ↑	↑↑	↑↑	↓	↓
AMRINONE	0	0	↑↑	↑	↓	↓
EPINEPHRINE	↑	↑↑	↑	0 to ↑	↓a ↑b	0 to ↓
NOREPINEPHRINE	↑↑	0 to ↓	0 to ↓	0 to ↑	↑	↑
DIGOXIN	0 to ↓	0 to ↓	↑	↑	=	↓
ISOPROTERENOL	↓	↑↑	↑↑	0 to ↓	↓	↓
DILTIAZEM (IV)	↓	0 to ↓	0 to ↑	0 to ↑	↓	=
NIFEDIPINE (IV)	↓↓	↑reflex	↑↑	=	↓↓↓	=
ACE INHIBITORS	↓	=	0 to ↑	↑↑	↓	↓↓
NITROGLYCERIN (IV)	↓	↑	↑	↑	↓	↓
Intra-Aortic balloon pump	↓	0	↑	↑	↓	↓

(a) slow infusion of epi   (b) rapid bolus of epi
↓- decrease, ↑ -increase, = - no change, multiple arrows - greater effect

GUIDELINES FOR PROPER SWAN-GANZ CATHETER PLACEMENT

CRITERION	ZONE 3	ZONE 1 or 2
PCWP CONTOUR	A & V waves present	Unnaturally smooth
PAD vs PCWP	PAD > PCWP	PAD < PCWP
PEEP TRIAL	ΔPCWP <½ ΔPEEP	ΔPCWP >½ ΔPEEP
RESPIRATORY VARIATION	<½ ΔP$_{ALV}$	≥½ ΔP$_{ALV}$
CATH TIP LOCATION	Below LA level	Above LA level

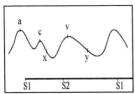

RA Waveformscomponents a wave- RA contracts; x descent – RA pressure ↓; c wave- RV begins contraction; v wave- RV ejection; y descent- tricuspid valve opens

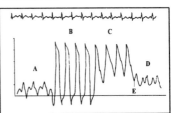

Pressure tracing: Swan-Ganz tip position in (A)Right atrium; (B) Right Ventricle; (C) Pulmonary Artery; (D) wedged with balloon inflated; (E) Point of balloon inflation

ABNORMALITIES OF VENTILATION
· Distribution disturbance
· Restrictive ventilation - *DDX*: Chest wall or respiratory muscle disorders (kyphoscoliosis, myasthenia gravis); Air space or parenchymal infiltrates (pulmonary edema, diffuse interstitial fibrosis); Pleura abnormalities (pleural thickening); Space occupying lesions (tumors, effusions, cardiac enlargement); Lung resection.
· Obstructive ventilation - *DDX*: Limitation of expiratory airflow (Asthma, bronchitis, emphysema, advanced bronchiectasis)
· Diffusion disturbance - *Decreased DL$_{CO}$ DDX*: Intra-alveolar filling process (blood, fluid, or pus); ↓ in both lung and blood components (lung resection, emphysema). ↑ *DL$_{CO}$ DDX*: Increase in capillary blood volume (↑ in pulmonary artery or Left atrial pressure, ex: CHF) OR (increased pulmonary blood flow, ex: ASD)
· Perfusion disturbance - measured with ^{135}I-albumin or ^{133}Xe in saline. *DDX*: emboli, vasculitis, emphysema, tumors, cysts, alveolar hypoxia with vasoconstriction.

PULMONARY FUNCTION TEST

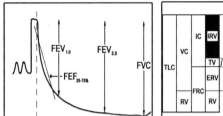
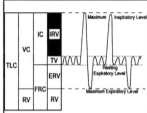

(TLC)Total Lung Capacity; (VC) Vital Capacity; (IC) Inspiratory Capacity; (TV) Tidal Volume; (FRC) Functional Residual Capacity; (IRV) Inspiratory Reserve Volume; (RV) Residual Volume; (ERV) Expiratory Reserve Volume; (FEV1) Forced Expiratory Volume in 1 sec; (FVC) Forced Vital Capacity; (FEF$_{25-75}$) Forced Expiratory Flow Slope between 25 & 75% of FVC.

5 CAUSES OF ARTERIAL HYPOXIA
- *Hypoventilation*: pure form is rare. *DDX*: Excess sedation, neuromuscular disease, COPD.
- *Impaired diffusion*: one of the major causes during exercise; not usually with rest. *DDX*:
  ↓vascular surface area, ↓ alveolar surface area, ↑ membrane thickness.
- *Ventilation-Perfusion* (V/Q) *mismatch*: MC cause of clinically encountered hypoxia; may have ↑ V/Q & ↓PO2 > ↑PCO2 with underventilated units; OR ↓ V/Q & ↑ PO2 & ↓PCO2 with underperfused units. *DDX*: Airway Dz., Interstitial Dz., Alveolar Dz., Pulm vascular Dz.
- *Right →Left shunting*: major cause of hypoxia during exercise; differentiate from V/Q mismatch with FIO2 of 100% & measure PaO2 after N2 washes out of lungs: V/Q mismatch will "correct" PaO2 to ≈600; R→L shunt the (A-a)O2 gradient actually worsens.
- *↓ inspired O2*: *DDX*: high altitude, ↓ FIO2.

INDICATIONS FOR INTUBATION
Airway Support
- Mechanical airway obstruction
- Pharyngeal instability
- Decreased LOC with absent gag reflex, absent cough, or inability to maintain airway with head in flexion
- Bulbar or generalized motor weakness

Miscellaneous
- Frequent recurrent non-perfusing arrhythmias
- Hemodynamically compromising sepsis

Respiratory Failure
- Tachypnea >35 breaths/min with accessory muscle recruitment & signs of patient distress (e.g., tachyarrhythmias or bradyarrhythmias, diaphoresis, severe dyspnea, clammy cyanosis)
- Severe uncompensated metabolic acidosis without an obviously reversible cause (pH<7.30)

TYPES OF VENTILATORS
•VOLUME-CYCLED
Controlled Mechanical Ventilation (CMV): Provides preset Rate & VT. Ventilatory pattern is continued independent of patient effort. Operator sets VT, rate, FIO2, inspiratory flow rate, wave form, PEEP, volume & ventilatory alarms. *Indications*: Pts. without spontaneous respirations. *Disadvantage*: If spontaneous respirations occur, may lead to Pt-ventilator desynchrony & aborted breaths due to high airway pressures.
Assist/Control (AC): "Assist" allows Pt. to initiate breaths. Ventilator provides full VT synchronized to Pt. effort. If Pt. fails to initiate breaths, then "Control" will deliver a breath within a predetermined cycle period. Operator sets backup "control" rate, inspiratory pressure threshold, VT, FIO2, inspiratory flow rate, wave form, PEEP, volume & ventilatory alarms. *Indications*: May be applied to awake, moderately sedated, or fully paralyzed Pts. *Disadvantage*: Tachypnea may lead to ventilator-assisted hyperventilation & respiratory alkalosis. COPD pts with tachypnea may develop auto-PEEP with potential for barotrauma.
Intermittent Mandatory Ventilation (IMV): Similar to CMV, except that pt. may spontaneously breath between mandatory breaths. Rate & VT of spontaneous breaths are determined by Pt.; supplementary mandatory breaths are determined by ventilator. *Indications*: Useful for weaning & conditioning of respiratory muscles. May be used as primary ventilation mode in Pt. with spontaneous respirations. *Disadvantages*: Ventilator-Pt. desynchrony can occur.

Synchronized IMV (SIMV): Similar to IMV, yet mandatory breaths are synchronized with Pt's respiratory pattern. (ie., Pt breathes spontaneously & when time for mandatory breath, ventilator waits predetermined time for pt. initiated breath. Any breath which occurs during this time period will be assisted by ventilator to preset VT; if no breath occurs, then ventilator delivers breath. *Disadvantage*: May provide less muscle conditioning than other modes of weaning. May add PSV to overcome this limitation.

Pressure Support Ventilation (PSV): Pt. triggered, flow-cycled pressure ventilation. Pt. initiates breath, ventilator supplies preset pressure at breath onset in square waveform until a minimum inspiratory flow rate is sensed. Rate & VT are determined by Pt. *Indications*: Primarily used for weaning. PSV is a more physiologic method of weaning as compared to SIMV.

•**HIGH-FREQUENCY JET VENTILATOR**: Non-conventional mode of ventilation where VT are dead space, & respiratory rates vary from 60-3600 bpm. Gas exchange occurs via bulk flow, gas flux, Taylor diffusion, non-convective mixing, & molecular diffusion. *Indications*: Hypoxia due to diffuse lung injury & persistent bronchopleural fistula. Has lower peak airway pressures & reduced FIO_2 requirements compared to other forms of ventilation. *Disadvantages*: Potential for gas trapping with secondary barotrauma, & necrotizing tracheobronchitis just down stream of the nozzle.

•**PRESSURE-CYCLED**: Delivery of a time cycled pressure wave; VT is dependent on respiratory system impedance; exhalation occurs passively. Several systems are modified to combine pt. triggering, pressure or flow cycling, with volume control backup. *Indications*: Same as volume cycled. Advantages include decelerating flow with lower peak airway pressures; also peak flow coincides with pt. maximal inspiratory effort. *Disadvantages*: Mainly that minute ventilation depends on respiratory impedance, & pt. with unstable respiratory mechanics must be observed closely.

•**NEGATIVE-PRESSURE**: Application of negative pressure to outer chest wall. (ex: iron lung)

•**POSITIVE END EXPIRATORY PRESSURE (PEEP)**: A fixed amount of positive pressure applied to a mechanical ventilation cycle when spontaneous breathing is not present.

•**CONTINUOUS POSITIVE-AIRWAY PRESSURE (CPAP)** :Same as PEEP, yet is term applied when spontaneous respirations are present. *Benefits*: potentially opens closed alveolar units, which ↑'s lung compliance and improves V/Q. *Indications*: to improve hypoxemia secondary to diffuse lung injury. It allows for lower FIO_2 to prevent O_2 toxicity.

WEANING PARAMETERS

•f/V$_T$	≤105 breaths/min/L	•Minute ventilation (V$_E$)	≤15 L/min
•Peak Negative Pressure .	≤-15 cm H_2O	•Resp Rate (f)	≤38 breaths/min
•Tidal Volume(V$_T$)	≥325 ml	•Static compliance (C$_{st}$)	≥33 ml/cm H_2O
•V$_T$/patient's wt	≥4 ml/kg	•PaO$_2$/PAO$_2$	≥0.35

(Yang KL, Tobin MJ. A Prospective Study of Indexes Predicting the Outcome of Trials of Weaning from Mechanical Ventilation. NEJM 1991; 324(21):1445-50.)

LACTIC ACID:
•Lactic Acid Normals: ≤ 2mEq/L OR ≤ 4mEq/L if stressed
•Increased Lactic Acid levels can be used to correlate the adequacy of therapies to increase tissue perfusion.
•DDX of increased Lactic Acid levels: ischemia, thiamine deficiency, bacterial pneumonia, generalized seizures, respiratory alkalosis, and generalized trauma.

HIGH OUTPUT FAILURE: DDX- Hyperthyroid, Beriberi, Paget's disease, A-V fistulas, emphysema, anemia

Critical Care Notes:

PRINCIPLES OF TOPICAL STEROID THERAPY

- The stratum corneum is the main barrier to absorption, so, diffusion is slow through thick skin such as the palms & soles, & faster through thin skin like the face, ears, & scrotum.
- The higher the concentration applied the greater the quantity absorbed.
- Creams are semisolid emulsions of oil in water that vanish when rubbed into the skin. They also contain preservatives that may be allergenic.
- Lotions are suspensions of powder in water that require shaking. Pruritus is relieved by the evaporation of the water that then leaves a light film of powder.
- Ointments are emulsions of water droplets that don't rub in. They are greasy, clear, & do not require preservatives. Use when hydration, occlusion, & maximal penetration are desired.

GUIDELINES FOR TOPICAL STEROID USE

- Begin with weak topical steroids for mild &/or chronic dermatoses which involve the face or intertriginous areas; never use fluorinated steroids on these areas.
- Use medium to strong topical steroids for more severe & recalcitrant dermatoses.
- Creams, Lotions, & Gels are used for acute or subacute inflammation with vesiculations & oozing. (Lotions & gels are best for hairy areas).
- Ointments (occlusive) are good for chronic inflammation with dryness, scaling, & lichenification, (ointments are less aesthetically acceptable, and they have ↓ potential for irritation & allergy.
- Frequency - the stratum corneum acts as a reservoir & continually releases steroid into the skin (usual dose QD-BID is sufficient). Note: *Tachyphylaxis* - when a potent steroid becomes less effective with chronic use.
- Amount guidelines: 1 gm ≈10 X 10cm area; Face ≈2 gm/application; Arm ≈3 gm/application; Leg ≈4 gm/application; Whole body ≈30 gm/application.
- Always start with the lower % of steroid, & ↑ when greater action is desired.

TOPICAL STEROID SIDE EFFECTS

- Skin atrophy with telangiectasia formation; or striae formation.
- Fluorinated steroids on the face can cause acne of the face or "perioral dermatitis."
- Promotion of dermatophytic fungal infections.
- Retarding wound & ulcer healing.
- Allergic contact dermatitis from vehicle, (suspect if rash gets worse with topical steroid).
- Uncommon: glaucoma, cataracts, & retarded corneal ulcer healing.
- Rare: Adrenal suppression, iatrogenic Cushing's syndrome, & growth retardation in children.

COMMON TOPICAL STEROIDS

(See *GUIDELINES FOR TOPICAL STEROID USE* above for dosing guidelines.) NF= non-fluorinated

Lowest potency

dexamethasone [Decadron Phosphate, Decaspray] 0.1% cream (15, 30 g), 0.01% (58 g) & 0.04% (25 g) aerosol
hydrocortisone acetate OTC [Cortaid] 0.5% cream, ointment (15, 30 g); 1% cream, ointment (15, 30 g)
hydrocortisone NF OTC [Cortizone 5] 0.5% cream (15, 30, 60 g), ointment (30 g); OTC [CortaGel] 0.5% gel (15, 30 g); OTC [Cortizone 10] 1.0% ointment (28, 30 g); OTC [Extra Strength CortaGel] 1% gel (15, 30 g); OTC [Maximum Strength Cortaid] 1% pump spray (45 ml)
hydrocortisone [Cetacort] 0.25% lotion (120 ml), 0.5% lotion (30, 60, 120 ml); [Hytone] 1% cream, ointment (15, 20, 30, 60, 120, 240 g); 1% lotion (60, 120 ml), solution (30, 60 ml); 2.5% cream (15, 20, 30, 60, 120, 240 g), ointment (20, 30 g), lotion (60, 120 ml)

Low potency

alclometasone dipropionate [Aclovate] 0.05% cream, ointment (tubes 15, 45, 60 g)
betamethasone valerate [Valisone] 0.01% cream (15, 60 g)
desonide [DesOwen, Tridesilon] 0.05% cream, ointment (15, 60 g), 0.05% lotion (60, 120 ml)
fluocinolone acetonide [Synalar] 0.01% cream (15, 30, 60 g), solution (20, 60 ml), shampoo (180 ml), oil (120 ml)
methylprednisolone acetate [Medrol Acetate Topical] 0.25%, 1% ointment (30 g)

Medium Potency

betamethasone benzoate [Uticort] 0.025% cream (60 g), gel (15, 60 g), lotion (60 ml)
betamethasone dipropionate [Diprosone] 0.05% lotion (20, 30, 60 ml)
betamethasone valerate [Valisone] 0.1% cream (15, 45 g); 0.1% lotion (20, 60 ml)
clocortolone pivalate [Cloderm] 0.1% cream (15, 45 g)
desoximetasone [Topicort LP] 0.05% cream (15, 60 g)
fluocinolone acetonide [Synalar] 0.025% cream, ointment (15, 30, 60 g)
flurandrenolide [Cordran, Cordran SP] 0.025% cream, ointment (30, 60 g); 0.05% cream, ointment (15, 30, 60 g); 0.05% lotion (15, 60 ml); 4 mcg/cm² tape (24"x3", 80"x3")

fluticasone propionate [Cutivate] 0.05% cream (15, 30, 60 g); 0.005% ointment (15, 60 g)
halcinonide [Halog] 0.025% cream (15, 60 g)
hydrocortisone buteprate [Pandel] 0.1% cream (15,45 g)
hydrocortisone valerate NF [Westcort] 0.2% cream (15, 45, 60, 120 g), ointment (15, 45, 60 g)
mometasone furoate [Elocon] 0.1% cream, ointment (15, 45 g), lotion (27.5, 55 ml)
triamcinolone acetonide [Aristocort A, Kenalog] 0.025% ointment (15, 80, 240 g), cream (15, 30, 60, 120, 240 g),
   lotion (60 ml); 0.1% ointment (15, 60, 80, 240 g), cream (15, 60, 80, 240 g), lotion (15, 60 ml); 0.5% ointment
   (15, 20, 240 g) cream (15, 30, 60, 120, 240 g); [Kenalog] aerosol (23, 63 g)

High Potency
amcinonide [Cyclocort] 0.1% cream, ointment (tubes 15, 30, 60 g), 0.1% lotion (20, 60 ml)
augmented betamethasone dipropionate [Diprolene] 0.05% cream, gel (15, 45 g), 0.05% lotion (30, 60 ml)
betamethasone dipropionate [Diprosone] 0.05% cream, ointment (15, 45 g), 0.1% aerosol (85 g)
betamethasone valerate [Valisone] 0.1% ointment (15, 45 g)
desoximetasone [Topicort] 0.05% gel (15, 60 g), 0.25% cream, ointment (15, 60, 120 g)
diflorasone diacetate [Florone, Maxiflor] 0.05% cream, ointment(emollient-based) (15, 30, 60 g)
fluocinolone acetonide [Synalar HP] 0.2% cream (12 g)
fluocinonide [Lidex, Lidex-E] 0.05% cream, ointment, gel (15, 30, 60, 120 g), & 0.05% solution (20, 60 ml)
halcinonide [Halog, Halog-E] 0.1% cream, ointment (15, 30, 60, 240 g); 0.1% solution (20, 60 ml)
triamcinolone acetonide [Delta-Tritex] 0.1% ointment (30 g)

Super-High Potency
augmented betamethasone dipropionate [Diprolene] 0.05% ointment (15, 45 g)
clobetasol propionate [Temovate] 0.05% cream, ointment (15, 30, 45, 60 g), 0.05% gel, emollient (15, 30, 60 g),
   0.05% scalp application (25, 50 ml)
diflorasone diacetate [Psorcon] 0.05% ointment (15, 30, 60 g)
halobetasol propionate [Ultravate] 0.05% cream, ointment (15, 45 g)

COMBINATION ANTI-INFECTIVES/CORTICOSTEROID
1+1-F Creme [3% clioquinol/1% pramoxine/1% hydrocortisone] cream (30 g)
Cortisporin [0.5% neomycin/10,000U polymyxin/0.5% hydrocortisone acetate] cream (7.5 g); [0.5%
   neomycin/400U bacitracin/5000U polymyxin/1% hydrocortisone] ointment (15 g)
Fungoid-HC [triacetin/cetyl Pyridium Cl/0.5% hydrocortisone] cream (30 g)
Lotrisone [1% clotrimazole/0.05% betamethasone dipropionate] cream (15, 45 g)
Myco-Biotic II [0.5% neomycin/100,000U nystatin/0.1% triamcinolone acetonide] cream (15, 30, 60 g)
Mycolog II [10,000U nystatin/0.1% triamcinolone] cream, ointment (15, 30, 60, 120 g)
Mytrex [10,000U nystatin/0.1% triamcinolone] cream, ointment (15, 30, 60 g)
Neo-Cortef [0.5% neomycin/1% hydrocortisone] cream (20 g); [0.5% neomycin/0.5% hydrocortisone acetate] &
   [0.5% neomycin/1% hydrocortisone acetate] ointment (20 g)
Neo-Medrol Acetate [0.5% neomycin/0.25% or 1% methylprednisolone] liquid (30 g)
Neo-Synalar [0.5% neomycin/0.025% fluocinolone] cream (15, 30, 60 g)
Neodecadron [0.5% neomycin/0.025% dexamethasone] cream (15, 30 g)
Vioform-Hydrocortisone [3% clioquinol/0.5% hydrocortisone] mild cream (15, 30 g); [3% clioquinol/1%
   hydrocortisone] cream (20, 30, 300 g); [3% clioquinol/1% hydrocortisone] ointment (20, 30 g)

MISCELLANEOUS CORTICOSTEROID COMBINATIONS
Carmol HC Cream [10% urea/1% hydrocortisone acetate] cream (30, 120 g)
Lida-Mantle-HC Cream [3% lidocaine/0.5% hydrocortisone acetate] cream (30 g)
Mantadil Cream [2% chlorcyclizine HCl/0.5% hydrocortisone acetate] cream (15 g)
Pramosone [1% pramoxine/1% hydrocortisone acetate] cream (30, 60, 120 g), ointment (30, 120 g), lotion (60,
   120, 240 ml); [1% pramoxine/2.5% hydrocortisone acetate] cream (30, 120 g), ointment (30, 120 g), lotion (60,
   120 ml)
ProctoCream-HC [1% pramoxine/1% hydrocortisone acetate] cream (30 g)
ProctoFoam-HC [1% pramoxine/1% hydrocortisone acetate] aerosol foam (10 g)
Vanoxide-HC [5% benzoyl peroxide/0.5% hydrocortisone] lotion (25 ml)
Vytone Cream [1% iodoquinol/1% hydrocortisone] cream (30 g)

TOPICAL ANTI-INFECTIVE AGENTS
acyclovir [Zovirax] 5% ointment (3, 15 g) apply 6 times daily for 7 days.
amphotericin B [Fungizone] 3% cream, ointment (20 g); 1% lotion (30 ml) BID/QID. *yeast*
A/T/S [2% erythromycin topical gel USP] 2% gel (30 g) apply QD/BID. *Acne vulgaris*
bacitracin OTC ointment (15, 30 g) QD-TID.
butenafine [Mentax] Cream 1% (2, 15, 30 g) Apply to affected area qd X 4wks. *interdigital tinea pedis*

chloramphenicol [Chloromycetin] 1% cream (30 g) TID/QID.
ciclopirox olamine [Loprox] 1% cream (15, 30, 90 g); 1% lotion (30 ml) BID. *fungal/yeast*
clotrimazole [Lotrimin, Mycelex] OTC 1% cream (12, 15 g), solution (10, 30ml); 1% lotion (30ml) BID. *fungal/yeast*
econazole [Spectazole] 1% cream (15, 30, 85 g) QD/BID. *fungal/yeast*
erythromycin 2% ointment (25 g); 2% gel (30, 60 g) QD-QID.
gentamicin [Garamycin] 0.1% cream, ointment (15 g) TID/QID.
haloprogin [Halotex] 1% cream (15, 30 g); 1% solution (10, 30 ml) BID. *fungal*
ketoconazole [Nizoral] 2% cream (15, 30, 60 g); 2% shampoo (120 ml) QD. *fungal/yeast*
mafenide [Sulfamylon] 85 mg/g cream (60, 120, 435 g) apply to burn QD-BID.
metronidazole [Noritate] (1% emollient cream) *Adults* apply thin film once daily after washing. *Rosacea*
miconazole [Monistat-Derm (R), Micatin (OTC)] 2% cream, powder, spray - BID. *fungal/yeast*
mupirocin [Bactroban, Bactroban Nasal] 2% ointment (1 g, 15 g tubes): ½ of 1 g tube each nostril BID X 5D.
naftifine HCl [Naftin] 1% cream, gel (15, 30, 60 g) apply cream QD, gel BID *fungal*
nitrofurazone [Furacin] 0.2% solution(pt, gal); 0.2% ointment(28, 56, 454g); 0.2% cream(28g) apply to burn QD.
Neosporin OTC [bacitracin/neomycin/polymyxin] (cream, ointment) 2-5 times daily.
nystatin [Mycostatin] R 100,000U/g cream, ointment, powder (15, 30 g) BID/TID. *yeast*
oxiconazole [Oxistat] 1% cream, lotion (30, 60 g) QD-BID. Fungal
penciclovir [Denavir] (10 mg/g cream) Apply q2° while awake X 4 days. *Herpes labialis*
Polysporin OTC [bacitracin/polymyxin] (ointment, aerosol, powder) 2-5 times daily.
povidone-iodine [Betadine] (ointment, liquid, solution, shampoo)
silver sulfadiazine [Silvadene, Flint] 1% cream (20, 50, 400, 1000 g) QD-BID to burns.
sulconazole [Exelderm] 1% cream (15, 30, 60 g); 1% solution (30 ml) QD-BID. *fungal*
terbinafine [Lamisil] (Cream 1% {15, 30 g}and Sol 1% in non-aerosol pump; Tab 250 mg) tinea pedis- AAA BID for 2 wk (cream)/ 1 wk (spray); tinea corporis/cruris- QD for 1 wk; tinea (pityriasis) versicolor- sol AAA BID for 1 wk; Onychomycosis: Fingernail – PO 250 mg/day for 6 weeks; Toenail – PO 250 mg/day for 12 weeks.
tolnaftate OTC [Tinactin] 1% cream, gel, solution, powder, aerosol powder & liquid - BID. *fungal*
triacetin [Fungoid] (solution, cream, tincture) cream/solution TID; tincture BID; [Ony-Clear Nail Spray] QD. *fungal*

LICE/SCABIES AGENTS

crotamiton [Eurax] (10% cream, lotion) total body neck down, repeat in 24h, bath after 48h. *scabies*
lindane R [Kwell, Scabene] (1% cream in 60 g; 1% lotion 30, 60 ml) apply total body neck down, wash off after 8-12h; (1% shampoo in 30, 60 ml) 30-60 cc per application, rinse after 4 min. *lice/scabies*
malathion [Ovide] (0.5% lotion in 59 ml) Sprinkle on dry hair, wash in 8-12h, may repeat in 7-10 days. *head lice*
permethrin [OTC: Nix 1% cream rinse] (60 ml bottle with comb) *Head lice* apply cream rinse to hair/scalp, rinse after 10 mins. [R Elimite 5% cream] (60 g tube) *Scabies* apply total body neck down, wash after 8-14h.
pyrethrins/piperonyl butoxide combinations OTC liquid, gel, shampoos) Refer to package insert.

ACNE PRODUCTS

adapalene [Differin] (Gel 0.1% (15, 45 g), Sol 1%) apply to affected areas once a day at bedtime after washing skin
A/T/S [2% erythromycin topical gel USP] 2% gel (30 g) apply QD/BID.
azelaic acid [Azelex] 20% Cream (30 g) acne- apply to affected areas twice daily after washing skin.
Benzamycin [30 mg erythromycin + 50 mg benzoyl peroxide/g of gel] (23.3 g) apply BID.
benzoyl peroxide OTC (5, 10% cleanser & cream; 5, 5.5, 10% lotion; 2.5, 5, 10% gel) wash or apply QD-BID.
erythromycin, topical 1.5% solution (60 ml); 2% solution (60, 120 ml) apply BID.
isotretinoin [Accutane] (10, 20, 40 mg tabs) 0.5-2 mg/kg/24h divided BID.
meclocycline sulfosalicylate, topical [Meclan] 1% cream (20, 45 g tube) apply BID.
metronidazole [MetroGel] 0.75% gel (30 g tube) wash, then apply thin film BID.
tazarotene [Tazorac] (Gel 0.05%, 0.1%) Apply thin film (2 mg/cm²) each evening to acne lesions.
tetracycline, topical [Topicycline] 2.2 mg/ml solution (70 ml) apply BID.
tretinoin [Retin-A] 0.025, 0.05, 0.1% cream (20,45 g);0.01, 0.025% gel (15,45 g); 0.05% liquid (28 ml), micronized 0.1% formula; apply HS

ENZYME PREPARATIONS, TOPICAL

collagenase [Santyl] (250 units/g) ointment (15, 30 g) apply once daily.
Elase [25U fibrinolysin/15,000U desoxyribonuclease per vial] lyophilized powder (30 ml vials); [1U fibrinolysin/666.6U desoxyribonuclease per gram] ointment (10, 30 g) per package insert.
Elase-Chloromycetin [10 mg chloramphenicol/1U fibrinolysin/666.6U desoxyribonuclease/g] ointment (10, 30 g)
Granulex [0.1 mg trypsin/72.5 mg Balsam Peru/650 mg castor oil per 0.87 ml] aerosol (60, 120 g) apply QD-BID.
Panafil [10% papain/10% urea/0.5% chlorophyllin copper] ointment (30 g) apply QD-BID.
sutilains [Travase] (82,000 casein units/g) ointment (14.2 g) apply 1/8" ointment 3-4 times daily.

CAUTERIZING AGENTS

<u>dichloroacetic acid</u> [Bichloracetic Acid] liquid (10 ml)
<u>monochloroacetic acid</u> [Monocete, Mono-Chlor] 80% liquid (15 ml)
<u>silver nitrate</u> 10% ointment (30 g); 10%, 25%, 50% solution (30 ml); 75% with 25% potassium nitrate applicators
<u>trichloroacetic acid</u> [Tri-Chlor] 80% liquid (15 ml)

MISCELLANEOUS DERMATOLOGICS

<u>acitretin</u> [Soriatane] (Cap 10, 25 mg) 25-50 mg QD with main meal. *Psoriasis*
<u>aluminum chloride hexahydrate</u> [Drysol] 20% solution (35, 37.5 ml) apply to affected area HS.
<u>amlexanox</u> [Aphthasol] (paste 5%) squeeze ≈0.25" of paste onto fingertip and apply to *aphthous ulcer*.
<u>ammoniated mercury</u> [Emersal] (Lotion 5% with 2.5% salicylic acid) *Psoriasis*- apply 1-2 times a day
<u>anthralin (dithranol)</u> [Drithocreme, Dritho-Scalp, Lasan] 0.1, 0.2, 0.25, 0.4, 0.5, 1% cream (50, 65 g); [Anthra-Derm, Lasan] 0.1, 0.25, 0.4, 0.5, 1% ointment (42.5, 60 g) Apply sparingly QD. *Psoriasis*
<u>becaplermin</u> [Regranex] (Gel 100 mcg) Apply QD to the diabetic ulcer until complete healing has occurred
<u>calamine</u> (lotion, cream, ointment, spray) apply TID-QID prn itching.
<u>calcipotriene</u> [Dovonex] (0.005% ointment) *Psoriasis* - apply thin layer BID, rub in gently & completely.
<u>cantharidin</u> [Verr-Canth] 0.7% liquid (7.5 ml) apply to wart with 1-3mm overlap, wash off after 24h.
<u>Cantharone Plus</u> [30% salicylic acid/2% podophyllum/1% cantharidin] liquid (7.5 ml).
<u>capsaicin</u> [Zostrix] 0.25% cream (45, 90 g), 0.75% cream (30, 60 g) to affected area not more than 3-4 times/d.
<u>chloroxine</u> [Capitrol] 2% shampoo (120 ml) apply shampoo, rinse after 3min, use twice weekly. *Seborrheic dermatitis*
<u>coal tar</u> OTC [Tegrin] apply shampoo daily.
<u>etretinate</u> [Tegison] (Tab 10, 25 mg) *Severe Recalcitrant Psoriasis* PO Initial 0.75-1 mg/kg/D in divided doses, Maintenance 0.5-0.75 mg/kg/D after 6-8 weeks. MAX 1.5 mg/kg/D
<u>finasteride</u> [Propecia] (Tab 1 mg) 1 mg QD
<u>hexachlorophene</u> ℞ [PhisoHex] 3% liquid soap (8 ml, 150 ml, pt, gal); [Septisol] 0.23% foam (180, 600 ml).
<u>hydroquinone</u> [Lustra] (cream 4%) Apply to affected areas BID. (1oz jar) *Depigmenting agent*
<u>imiquimod</u> [Aldara] 0.5% Cream (250 mg packets) Apply 3 times weekly HS & leave on for 6-10 hours. MAX 16wks. *genital & perianal warts*
<u>masoprocol</u> [Actinex] 10% cream (30 g) apply to affected area BID
<u>mefenide</u> [Sulfamylon] (sol 5%, cream 85 mg/g) Apply to the clean and debrided wound with a sterile gloved hand, once or twice daily, to a thickness of approximately 1/16 inch. Adjunctive therapy of second and third degree burns.
<u>methionine</u> (200 mg cap; 500 mg tab; 75 mg/5 ml liquid) *Diaper rash* use 75 mg in warm formula TID-QID; *Incontinent adult odor control* use 200-500 mg TID-QID.
<u>methotrexate</u> (Tab 2.5 mg; 25 mg/ml inj) *Psoriasis* 10-25 mg IM/IV q wk; 2.5 mg PO q12h for 3 doses. MAX 30 mg/wk.
<u>minoxidil</u> [Rogaine] 20 mg/ml solution (60 ml) apply 1 ml to dry scalp BID.
<u>monobenzone</u> [Benoquin] 20% cream (35.4 g) apply to pigmented areas BID-TID.
<u>oatmeal</u> [Aveeno] apply lotion QID prn itching.
<u>podofilox</u> [Condylox] 0.5% solution, gel (3.5 ml) *Warts* apply BID X 3d, stop X 4d, then repeat 4 more times
<u>podophyllum resin</u> [Pod-Ben-25] (25% podophyllum in tincture of benzoin) liquid (15, 30 ml) physician applied
<u>selenium sulfide</u> [Selsun] (2.5% in 120 ml) shampoo, rinse after 2-3min, 2-7 times weekly.
<u>sulfacetamide sodium</u> [Sebizon] (10% lotion in 85 g) apply HS, leave on overnight. *Seborrheic dermatitis*.
<u>Verrex</u> [30% salicylic acid/10% podophyllum] liquid (7.5 ml with applicator).
<u>Verrusol</u> [30% salicylic acid/5% podophyllum/1% cantharidin] liquid (7.5 ml).

Dermatology Notes:

TRAUMA SURVEY PRIMARY SURVEY: "ABCDE", Solve Life Threatening problems as you discover them!

AIRWAY & C-SPINE - Assess and perform required actions (i.e. ET or NT intubation) to obtain and maintain a patent airway while sustaining C-spine control. Immobilize neck if C-spine injury is suspected. Possible interventions: 1)Chin lift, 2)Insert oral or nasal airway, 3)Obtunded or unconscious pt.- should ET or NT intubate to protect airway and hyperventilate, 4)Paralyzing agent for the very agitated pt.

BREATHING- Assess breath sounds (BS), trachea position and chest wall (ie flail chest, sucking chest wound or subcutaneous air). 100% O_2 if pt has spontaneous respirations. Possible interventions: 1)Unequal BS- withdraw ET tube from Right mainstem or reintubate if no BS, 2)Deviated trachea- insert needle into chest to relieve tension pneumothorax, 3)Sucking chest wound- apply occlusive dressing as pt breaths out, 4)Chest tube placement, 5)Thoracotomy- ie large hemothorax.

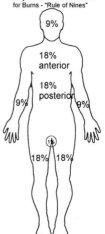

Body Surface area estimation for Burns - "Rule of Nines"

9%
18% anterior
18% posterior
9% 9%
1%
18% 18%
9% 9%

CIRCULATION - Check pulses (palpable carotid then BP ≈60, palpable femoral then BP ≈70, palpable radial then BP ≈80).Quality of heart tones- clear or distant (tamponade). Possible interventions: 1)Rapid infusion of crystalloid if no pulse or no marked improvement after 2L use O neg PRBCs, 2)Direct pressure to any exsanguinating hemorrhages.

DISABILITY-Level of consciousness: **A**lert, Response to **V**ocal stimuli, **P**ainful stimuli or **U**nresponsive.

EXPOSURE AND VITALS- Maintain stable spine, undress, complete visual exam.

RESUSCITATION

O_2, monitor, Start IV's. Get initial lab: blood type & cross (Shock: 2 units, plus 2 units for every 40 mmHg ↓ in normal systolic BP; decreased HCT- <30%: 2 units; Observed EBL > 500ml or gross GI bleed: 2 units; OR: 2 units for each liter of anticipated blood loss), ABG, CBC, SMA7.

SECONDARY SURVEY: "Fingers or Tubes in every opening". Perform after stabilizing life threatening problems. Complete examination from head to toe.

HEAD: Lacerations, other trauma. ALL head trauma patients should be properly observed, especially after loss of consciousness, for possible delayed intracranial complications- "ALWAYS THINK BLEEDS"!!

EYES: pupils, fundi, acuity. **EARS**: fluid, blood. **NOSE**: CSF, septum.

NECK: cross-table, open mouth & AP C-spine X-ray. NG or OG tube prn

CHEST: Get CXR. R/O aortic, tracheobronchial, esophageal, and diaphragmatic disruption, pulmonary contusion

PELVIS: Palpate bony pelvis. Urethral meatus for blood, if present DO NOT catheterize!

RECTAL: Examine prostate. Blood? Check sphincter tone.

NEURO: COMPLETE EXAM with emphasis on pupils, fundi, reflexes and level of consciousness.

ANAPHYLAXIS:℞ Mild: Epinephrine 1:1,000SQ, PEDS: 0.01mg/kg, ADULTS: 0.3-0.5 ml

BURNS: DEGREE: 1°-Erythema & pain; 2°- Blisters, edema, increased pain, erythema; 3°-Full thickness, charred, dark or white, painless. AREA: "Rule of Nines"-Head 9%, Arm 9%, Chest 18%, Back 18%, Leg 18%, Genitalia 1% (see above) FLUIDS: LR 4cc/kg/%burn, give 50% 1st 8h then 50% next 16h.

COMA: ABC's:•O_2 Tracheal intubation. IV access. History available?
•Lab-STAT glucose, lytes, calcium, ABG, ethanol level, toxicology screen, CBC, cultures, UA
•Give 50ml of D_{50} IV (if hypoglycemic by FSBS) and thiamine 100mg IV•naloxone [Narcan] (0.2, 0.4 & 1.0 mg/ml) IM/IV 5-10 mcg/kg/dose q 3-5 min prn. MAX 2mg
•consider- flumazenil [Romazicon] IV 0.2 mg over 30sec then 0.3-0.5 mg q30 sec prn, MAX 3mg
•consider CT, lumbar puncture, EEG, liver and thyroid profile

DDX: Drugs, alcohol, hypoxia, infection, hypoglycemia, bleed, trauma, hypo- or hyperthermia, hypertensive encephalopathy, postictal state, tumor, myxedema, uremia, hepatic failure, other metabolic derangements.

GLASGOW COMA SCALE (Prognostic indicator: GCS of 3-4 has 85% chance of dying or remaining vegetative)

Eyes[1] open:		Verbal[2] response:		Motor[3] response:	
Spontaneously	4	Oriented & conversant	5	Obeys verbal command	6
To verbal command	3	Disoriented & conversant	4	To painful stimulus:	
To pain	2	Inappropriate words	3	Localizes painful stimulus	5
No response	1	Incomprehensible sounds	2	Flexion or withdrawal	4
		No response	1	Decorticate rigidity	3
				Decerebrate rigidity	2
Scale 3-15				No response	1

[1]Spontaneous eye opening suggests intact reticular activating system. [2]Conversant means well articulated & organized speech. This indicates a relatively intact CNS. [3]Most important & reproducible. No response suggests medullary involvement or a concomitant spinal cord injury.

NARCOTICS OVERDOSE: Naloxone PEDS:0.01-0.02mg/kg IV/IM, ADULTS: 2.0mg IV/ IM
PEDIATRIC FEVERS: see antimicrobials in Pediatrics Chapter

SHOCK-HEMORRHAGIC:

SHOCK CLASS	CLINICAL		BLOOD LOSS		MENTAL STATUS	FLUID
	PULSE	BP	%	MI		
I	<100	NORMAL	<15	<750	Agitated	RINGERS
II	>100		15-30	750-1500		
III	>120	↓	30-40	1500-2000	Anxious Confused Lethargic	RINGERS OR BLOOD
IV	>140		>40	>2000		

ASTHMA EXACERBATION:

Severity Classification	Resp Rate	Pulse	Pulsus Paradoxus	Breathless while	Alertness	PEF% SaO₂%
Mild	↑	<100	<10 mmHg	Walking	May be agitated	80 / >95
Moderate	↑	100-120	10-25	Talking	Likely agitated	50-80 / 91-95
Severe	↑↑ >30	>120	>25	At rest	Agitated	<50 / <91
Arrest imminent		<60	Absent		Drowsy or confused	

Treatment of Acute Asthma Exacerbation
- History and physical exam, PEF, O₂ saturation, Oxygen to achieve O₂ saturation ≥ 90%
- <u>PEF or FEV₁≥ 50%</u>
- inhaled β2 agonist by MDI or nebulizer; up to 3 doses in the first hour
- oral systemic corticosteroid if no immediate response or if patient recently took oral steroid
  - <u>PEF or FEV₁ remains 50-80%</u>- continue nebulizer β2 agonist treatments every hour for 1-3 hours
    - Incomplete response- PEF or FEV₁ ≥ 50 < 70%- individualized decision to admit or discharge
    - Good response- PEF or FEV₁ ≥ 70% sustained 1 hour after last treatment - discharge to home; continue inhaled β2 agonist by MDI; course of oral systemic corticosteroids; close medical follow up
- <u>PEF or FEV₁ < 50%</u>
- inhaled high dose β₂ agonist and anticholinergic q 20 min or continuous for 1 hour
- oral systemic corticosteroid
  - <u>PEF or FEV₁ remains < 50%</u>- continue nebulizer treatments hourly or continuously
    - Poor response- PEF or FEV₁ remains < 50%- admit to hospital for nebulizer treatments hourly or continuous, IV corticosteroids
    - Incomplete response- PEF or FEV₁ ≥ 50 < 70%- individualized decision to admit or discharge
    - Good response- PEF or FEV₁ ≥ 70%- discharge to home; continue inhaled β₂ agonist by MDI; course of oral systemic corticosteroids; close medical follow up
- Impending Respiratory arrest
- intubation and mechanical ventilation, inhaled high dose β₂ agonist and anticholinergic
- admit to hospital

WOUND MANAGEMENT
<u>LOCAL ANESTHETIC</u>: Don't use local anesthetic with Epinephrine on "Fingers, Toes, Nose and Penis".
<u>lidocaine</u> [Xylocaine] Nerve block 0.5%, 1%, 1.5%, 2% with or without epi; Maximum doses of Xylocaine: without epinephrine 4.5 mg/kg, with epi 7 mg/kg; 1% Xylocaine is 10 mg/ml, 2% Xylocaine is 20 mg/ml (Amide class)
<u>procaine</u> [Novocaine] Local 1.0% Maximum doses: without epinephrine 7 mg/kg, with epi 9 mg/kg (Ester class)
See Anesthetic section in Neurology chapter for more details.
May buffer lidocaine buffer with sodium bicarbonate 1 ml of 1 mEq/ml added to 10 ml lidocaine. Store in dark, refrigerator for up to 2 weeks. Warmed to room temp before use.
<u>SUTURES</u>: Face- 5-0 & 6-0 nylon or prolene. Scalp and trunk 3-0 and 4-0 nylon or prolene. Deep tissue-absorbable sutures (Vicryl, Dexon) 3-0 and 4-0. DO NOT (Routinely) SUTURE: human bites, animal bites, missile wounds, dirty or contaminated wounds or wounds >8 hours old. Keep covered with protective, nonadherent dressing for at least 24-48 hours. Should be kept clean and gently cleansed after 24-48 hours Remove after 10-14 days if subject to large tension forces, 7-12 days on extremities, 7 days scalp and body, and 3-5 days on face.

SKIN ADHESIVES:

octyl cyanoacrylate [Dermabond] (sterile, single-use ampule) manually crush the inner glass portion of the ampule, paint the adhesive on top of the skin as the laceration is manually approximated, apply at least 3 or 4 coats.★ Patients may shower, but avoid bathing and swimming. Avoid picking, scrubbing or prolonged exposure to water. Will usually slough off in 7 days.

TETANUS PROPHYLAXIS:

Clean, Minor Wounds- Tetanus and Diphtheria toxoid(Td) if > 10yrs since last dose, history of <3 Td doses or unknown. Diphtheria and Tetanus toxoid and Pertussis vaccine for children <7yrs that have not completed the series.

All Other Wounds- Tetanus and Diphtheria toxoid(Td) if > 5yrs since last dose, history of <3 Td doses or unknown. Diphtheria and Tetanus toxoid and Pertussis vaccine for children <7yrs that have not completed the series. Tetanus immune globulin [Hyper-Tet] if status of active immunization with tetanus toxoid is uncertain.

Emergency Medicine Notes:

DIABETES MELLITUS

Diagnosis and Classification of Diabetes Mellitus	
Normal Fasting Plasma Glucose ≤ 110 mg/dl	
Impaired glucose metabolism (or impaired glucose homeostasis)	
Impaired Fasting Glucose (IFG)	fasting plasma glucose is ≥ 110 but < 126 mg/dl
Impaired Glucose Tolerance (IGT)	oral glucose tolerance test are ≥140 but < 200 mg/dl (in the two-hour sample)
Diabetes Mellitus	
Diabetes can be diagnosed in any one of the following three ways, confirmed on a different day by repeating any one of these three tests:	
FPG **(preferred test)** of ≥126 mg/dl (after fasting for at least 8 hours); or	
Casual plasma glucose (taken at any time of day without regard to time of last meal) ≥ 200 mg/dl with the classic diabetes symptoms of increased urination, increased thirst and unexplained weight loss; or Oral glucose tolerance test (OGTT) value of ≥200 mg/dl in the two-hour sample.	

Diabetes Care 20:7 July 1997

DIABETIC MEDICATIONS

INSULIN 100 units/ml, 10 ml vials, NPH= isophane susp, Lente= zinc susp, Ultralente= extended zinc susp, DNA= human recombinant DNA, B&P= beef and pork, HSS= human semi-synthetic

Humalog [lispro] (DNA) [100u/ml in 10ml vials and 1.5 ml cartridges] SC, new rapid onset, Onset ≈15 min, Peak ≈0.5-1hr, Duration ≈2-3hrs

Humulin L [lente] (DNA) SC, dose as directed. Onset 1-3hrs, Peak 6-12hrs, Duration 18-24hrs

Humulin N [NPH] (DNA) SC, dose as directed. Onset 1-2hrs, Peak 6-12hrs, Duration 18-24hrs

Humulin R [Reg] (DNA) SC/IM/IV, dose as directed. Onset 30min, Peak 2-4hrs, Duration 6-8hrs

Humulin U [ultralente] (DNA) SC, dose as directed. Onset 4-6hrs, Peak 8-20hrs, Duration 24-28hrs

Humulin 70/30 [NPH 70%/Reg 30%] (DNA) SC, dose as directed. Onset 30min, Peak 2-12hrs, Duration 24 hrs

Humulin 50/50 [NPH 50%/Reg 50%] (DNA) SC, dose as directed. Onset 30min, Peak 3-5hrs, Duration 24 hrs

Iletin I Lente (B&P) SC, dose as directed. Onset 1-3hrs, Peak 6-12hrs, Duration 18-24hrs

Iletin I NPH (B&P) SC, dose as directed. Onset 1-2hrs, Peak 6-12hrs, Duration 18-26hrs

Iletin I Reg (B&P) SC/IM/IV, dose as directed. Onset 30min, Peak 2-4hrs, Duration 6-8hrs

Iletin I Semilente (B&P) SC, dose as directed. Onset 1-2hrs, Peak 3-8hrs, Duration 12-16hrs

Iletin I Ultralente (B&P) SC, dose as directed. Onset 4-6hrs, Peak 14-24hrs, Duration 28-36hrs

Iletin II Lente (purified B&P) SC, dose as directed. Onset 1-3hrs, Peak 6-12hrs, Duration 18-24hrs

Iletin II NPH (purified B&P) SC, dose as directed. Onset 1-2hrs, Peak 6-12hrs, Duration 18-26hrs

Iletin II Reg (purified B&P) SC/IM/IV, dose as directed. Onset 30min, Peak 2-4hrs, Duration 6-8hrs

Insulatard NPH Human (HSS) SC, dose as directed. Onset 1.5hrs, Peak 4-12hrs, Duration 24hrs

Insulatard NPH (purified Pork) SC, dose as directed. Onset 1.5hrs, Peak 4-12hrs, Duration 24hrs

Insulin Purified Lente (purified Pork) SC, dose as directed. Onset 2.5hrs, Peak 7-15hrs, Duration 22hrs

Insulin Purified NPH (purified Pork) SC, dose as directed. Onset 1.5hrs, Peak 4-12hrs, Duration 24hrs

Insulin Purified R [Reg] (purified Pork) SC/IM/IV, dose as directed. Onset 0.5hrs, Peak 2.5-5hrs, Duration 8hrs

Insulin NPH (Beef) SC, dose as directed. Onset 1.5hrs, Peak 4-12hrs, Duration 24hrs

Insulin R [Reg] (Pork) SC/IM/IV, dose as directed. Onset 0.5hrs, Peak 2.5-5hrs, Duration 8hrs

Mixtard 70/30 [NPH 70%/Reg 30%] (purified Pork) SC, dose as Mixtard Human 70/30

Mixtard Human 70/30 [NPH 70%/Reg 30%] SC, dose as directed. Onset 30min, Peak 4-8hrs, Duration 24hrs

Novolin L [lente] (DNA) SC, dose as directed. Onset 2.5hrs, Peak 7-15hrs, Duration 22hrs

Novolin N [NPH] (DNA) SC, dose as directed. Onset 1.5hrs, Peak 4-12hrs, Duration 24hrs

Novolin R [Reg] (DNA) SC/IM/IV, dose as directed. Onset 30min, Peak 2-4hrs, Duration 8hrs

Novolin 70/30 [NPH 70%/Reg 30%] (DNA) SC, dose as directed. Onset 30min, Peak 2-12hrs, Duration 24 hrs

Semilente (Beef) SC, dose as directed. Onset 1.5hrs, Peak 5-10hrs, Duration -16hrs

Velosulin [Reg] (purified Pork) SC/IM/IV, dose as directed. Onset 30min, Peak 1-3hrs, Duration 8hrs

Velosulin Human BR [Reg](semi-synthetic)SC/IM/IM,dose as directed. Onset 30min, Peak 1-3hrs,Duration 8hrs

ORAL GLUCOSE LOWERING AGENTS (O=onset & D=duration in hours, G=first or second generation Sulfonylureas, AL= alpha-glucosidase inhibitor, ME= meglitinide, TH= thiazolidinedione). CI in pregnancy.

acarbose [Precose] (Tab 50, 100 mg) Begin with 25 mg TID with the first bite of each meal (may start with once a day and 'if GI side effects tolerated); Increase to 50 mg (≤60kg) or 100 mg (≥ 60kg) TID as needed. AL

acetohexamide [Dymelor] [Tab 250, 500 mg] PO initial dose 250-1000 mg/d, doses >1gm/d should be divided BID, MAX 1.5gm/d. O=1, D=12-24, G=1 chlorpropamide [Diabinese] (Tab 100, 250 mg) PO initially 250 mg, adjust by 50-100 mg in 3-5 d intervals, maintenance 100-500 mg QD. MAX 750 mg/d. O=1, D=up to 60, G=1

glimepiride [Amaryl] (Tab 1, 2, 4mg) initial dose 1-2mg QD with breakfast, maintenance 1-4mg QD. Max 8mg/d. O=2-3, D=up to 24, G=2

glipizide [Glucotrol, XL] (Tab 2.5, 5, 10 mg) PO initially 5 mg 30 min before breakfast, ↑ by 2.5-5 mg q3-4 days, Max 15 mg single dose or 40 mg/d in divided dose. MAX 20 mg/d. O=1-1.5, D=10-16, G=2. XL 5-10 mg QD,

glyburide [Diabeta, Micronase, {Glynase PresTab}] (Tab 1.25, {1.5, 3}, 2.5, 5 mg) PO initially 2.5-5 mg QD with breakfast, ↑ weekly by 2.5 mg, usual maintenance 1.25-20 mg QD or divided BID, MAX 20 mg/d; Glynase presTab 1.5-3 mg/d with breakfast initial dose, then 0.75-12mg/d in single or divided doses. O=2-4, D=24, G=2

metformin [Glucophage] (Tab 500, 850mg) initially 500mg BID or 850mg QD, ↑ by 500mg q week or 850mg q other week given BID. Dose >2000mg/d give TID; Max 2550mg/d. Contraindicated in renal insufficiency.

miglitol [Glyset] (Tab 25, 50, 100mg) Initial 25 mg PO TID with first bite of meal, increase to 100 mg TID as needed for glycemic control. AL

pioglitazone [Actos] (Tab 15, 30, 45 mg) PO 15-30mg Q D, may increase up to 45 mg QD; mono or combo therapy. TH ★

repaglinide [Prandin](Tab 0.5, 1, 2 mg) PO 0.5 to 4 mg taken before or with meals, stimulates insulin release from pancreas. ME

rosiglitazone [Avandia] (Tab 2, 4, 8 mg) initially 4mg daily, may increase to 8 mg daily after 12 weeks. TH ★

tolazamide [Tolinase] (Tab 100, 250, 500 mg) PO 100-250 mg QD with breakfast, adjust 100-250 mg weekly, maintenance 0.1-1gm, doses >500 mg should be divided BID. O=4-6, D=12-24, G=1

tolbutamide [Orinase] (Tab 250,500mg) PO 1-2gm QD, maintenance 0.25-3gm QD or ÷ BID. O=1,D=6-12,G=1

troglitazone [Rezulin] (Tab 200,400 mg) PO start with 200 mg QD with a meal (continue current insulin dose; ↓ insulin 12-25% when fasting glucose is < 120 mg/dl); ↑after 2-4 wks if needed. MAX 600 mg/d. TH

GLUCOSE ELEVATING AGENTS

diazoxide [Proglycem] (Tab 50 mg Elx 50 mg/ml) PO 3-8 mg/kg/D divided BID/TID

glucagon IM/IV 0.5-1 mg, may be repeated in 15min if needed

glucose [B-D Glucose] (Tab 5gm) PO 10-20 gm, may repeat in 10 minutes

FERTILITY AGENTS

Clomid [clomiphene] (Tab 50 mg) PO 50 mg QD for 5 days

The following 3 drugs are used in polycystic ovary syndrome with HCG to induce ovulation and in Assisted Reproductive Technologies to induce multiple follicles:

follitropin alfa [Gonal-F] (Inj 75, 150 IU) see package insert for dosing

follitropin alfa [Follistim] (Inj 75 IU) see package insert for dosing

urofollitropin [Fertinex] (Inj 75, 150 IU) see package insert for dosing

MINERALS / VITAMINS

ascorbic acid [vitamin C] (Tab 25, 50, 100, 250, 500, 1000 mg) PO 50-250 mg QD

Beelith [magnesium/pyridoxine] (Tab 362mg/20mg) PO 1 tab QD

calcitriol [Rocaltrol, Calcijex] (Cap 0.25, 0.5 mcg; Sol 1 mcg/ml; Inj 1, 2 mcg/ml) initially 0.25 mcg QD, may increase by 0.25 mcg to 2 mcg/day at 4-6 week intervals.

calcium carbonate [Os-Cal] (Tab 500 mg) PO 0.25-3gm QD

calcium carbonate + Vit D [Os-Cal+D] (Tab 250, 500 mg) PO 0.5-2gm BID/TID/QID

calcium chloride (1000mg/10ml) Slow IV 0.1-1g

calcium gluconate (Tab 500mg, Inj 1000mg/10ml) PO 500-1000 mg BID/QID, Slow IV 0.1-1g

Caltrate 600+Iron & Vit D [calcium carbonate 600 mg, iron 18 mg, vit D 125 IU] PO 1-2 tabs QD

cyanocobalamin [Vit B12] (Tab 25, 50, 100, 250 μg) PO 25-100 μg, up to 1000 μg/d; IM/SC 100-200 μg q mo

dihydrotachysterol [Vit D, DHT] (Tab 0.125, 0.2, 0.4 mg Sol 0.2mg/ml) PO 0.2-1 QD

Ferrlecit [Sodium Ferric Gluconate Complex 62.5 mg elemental iron/5 ml] iron deficiency in chronic hemodialysis patients on supplemental erythropoetin therapy ★

ferrous gluconate 11.6% elemental iron (Cap 86;{Tab 300,320,325 mg; Elx 300mg/5ml) Dose- see ferrous sulfate

ferrous sulfate 20% elemental iron (Cap 250; Tab 195, 300, 324, 525 mg; Elx 220mg/5ml; Drop 75/0.6ml, 25/ml) PO Adults 100-200 mg (2-3 mg/kg) elemental iron daily divided TID - usual therapeutic dose. Children 2-12 yr 3mg/kg/D, 6 mo-2yr 6mg/kg/D; infants 10-25mg/D divided in 3-4 doses

folic acid [Folvite] (Tab 0.1, 0.4, 0.8, 1 mg) PO/SC/IM/IV 0.4-1 mg QD

Iberet-Folic-500 [ferrous sulfate 105 mg, ascorbic acid 500 mg, thiamine 6 mg, folic acid 0.8 mg, calcium 10 mg, cyanocobalamin 0.25 mg, pyridoxine 5 mg, riboflavin 6 mg] PO 1 tab QD

K-Phos M.F. & No.2 [potassium phosphate (mg)/sodium phosphate (mg)] (Tab M.F 155/350, No.2 305/700) PO M.F.- 2 QID; No.2- 1 QID with full glass of water.

K-Phos Neutral [phosphorus 250 mg, sodium 298 mg{13 mEq}, potassium 45 mg{1.1 mEq}] PO 1-2 QID with glass of water

levocarnitine [Carnitor] (Tab 330mg; Cap 250mg; Sol 100mg/ml)PO Sol 1-3g/d; Tab 990mg bid/tid; IV 50mg/kg
magnesium gluconate [Magonate] (Tab 500 mg Liq 54mg/5ml) PO 54-483mg/d in divided doses
magnesium hydroxide [Maalox] (magnesium hydroxide 200mg/aluminum hydroxide 200mg) PO 1-4 tabs QID
magnesium sulfate IV 2g in NS 100cc over 20 min, IM 1g q6h PRN
Mag-Ox 400 [magnesium oxide] (Tab 400 mg) OTC PO 1-2 tabs QD
Magtab SR [magnesium lactate] (Tab 84 mg {7 mEq}) OTC PO 1-2 tabs BID
Megadose [MVI] PO 1 tab QD
multivitamins [OTC] PO 1 tab QD, IV 1 amp in TPN or in NS/D5NS 500-1000cc
niacin [vitamin B3] (Tab 25, 50, 100, 250, 500 mg) PO 10-20 mg QD
omega-3-fatty acid [Promega] (Tab 600, 1000, 1200 mg) PO 1-2 tabs TID with meals
potassium bicarbonate [K-Lyte, K-Lyte DS] (effervescent Tab 25, 50 mEq) PO 1 tab in solution as directed
potassium chloride [K-Dur] (Tab 10, 20 mEq) PO 1-2 tabs QD, or as needed for replacement.
potassium gluconate [Kolyum liq] (Liq 20 mEq/15ml) PO doses as needed
pyridoxine [vitamin B6] (Tab 25, 50, 100 mg) PO 10-20 mg QD for 3 wks for deficiency
retinol [vitamin A] (Drp 5000IU/0.1ml Tab 10,000, 25,000, 50,000 IU) PO 5,000 IU QD
riboflavin [vitamin B2] (Tab 25, 50, 100 mg) PO 5-25 mg QD
sodium polystyrene sulfonate [Kayexalate] PO Suspension 15-60g QD; 15g 1- 4 times QD; *Children* 1 g/kg q6h;
    Powder mix in 20-100 ml water, or in sorbitol to prevent constipation; Enema (less effective) 30-50g q6h in 50-
    100 ml of fluid , retention for 30 min.
Slow-Mag [535 mg magnesium chloride hexahydrate (64 mg magnesium)] OTC Dietary supplement- 54-483
    mg/day in divided doses; RDAs- Males, 350-400 mg; females, 280-300 mg ★
thiamine [vitamin B1] (Tab 50, 100, 250, 500 mg) PO/IM/IV 100 mg QD
tocopherol [vitamin E, E-Gems] (Tab 30, 100, 200, 400, 600, 800, 1000, 1200IU) PO 30 IU QD
Uro-Mag [magnesium oxide 140 mg] PO 1 tab QD, Max 4 tabs a day for 2 weeks
Vicon Forte [vit A, B1, B2, B3, B6, B12, C, E and Ca, Mg, Zn] PO 1 tab QD
vitamin K [AquaMEPHYTON, Mephyton Tabs] (Tab 5 mg) PO/SC/IM 2.5-10 mg up to 25 mg
zinc sulfate (Tab 66, 110, 200, 220 mg) PO 25-50 mg QD supplement

CORTICOSTEROIDS

Generic Name	Equivalent Doses & Relative Potencies of Corticosteroids			
	Relative Anti-inflammatory	Relative Na+ Retaining	Equivalent Dose (mg)	Duration of Action (hr)
Betamethasone	25	0	0.75	36-72
Cortisol	1	1	20	8-12
Cortisone	0.8	0.8	25	8-12
Dexamethasone	25	0	0.75	36-72
Fludrocortisone	10	125		8-12
Methylprednisolone	5	0.5	4	12-36
Paramethasone	10	0	2	36-72
Prednisolone	4	0.8	5	12-36
Prednisone	4	0.8	5	12-36
Triamcinolone	5	0	4	12-36

betamethasone [Celestone] (Tab 0.6mg; Syp 0.6mg/5ml) PO 0.6-7.2mg QD; IV/IM Na+ phosphate; MAX 9mg/d
cortisone [Cortone] (Tab 5, 10, 25 mg) PO 25-300 mg QD
dexamethasone [Decadron] (Elx 0.5 mg/5ml Tab 0.25, 0.5, 0.75, 1, 1.5, 2, 4, 6mg) PO 0.75-9mg/d
dexamethasone acetate [Decadron-LA] IM 8-16 mg q1-3 weeks
dexamethasone sodium phosphate [Decadron Phosphate] IM/IV 0.5-9 mg/d divided q6-12h
fludrocortisone [Florinef] (Tab 0.1 mg) PO 0.1 mg QD *Addison disease*
flunisolide [Nasalide] (1 spray = 25µg) Nasal 2 sprays BID/TID
hydrocortisone [Cortef, Solu-Cortef] (Susp 10mg/5ml Tab 5,10,20mg) PO 20-240mg/d; IM/IV 100-500mg q4-6h
methylprednisolone [Medrol] (Tab 2, 4, 8, 16, 24, 32 mg) PO 4-48 mg QD
methylprednisolone sodium succinate [Solu-Medrol] IM/IV 10-40 mg q8h or high dose 30 mg/kg IV q4-6h
prednisolone [Prelone Liq] (Liq 5, 15 mg/5ml; Tab 5 mg) PO 5-60 mg QD
prednisolone sodium phosphate IM/IV 4-60mg/d
prednisone [Deltasone, Liq Pred] (Elx 5 mg/5ml; Tab 1, 2.5, 5, 10, 20, 50 mg) PO 5-60 mg QD or 1-2mg/kg/d
triamcinolone [Aristocort, Kenacort] (Syp 4mg/5ml; Tab 1, 2, 4, 8 mg) PO 4-48 mg QD
triamcinolone diacetate IM 40 mg q week

SEX STEROIDS (✱therapy may be given continuous in patient who does not have an uterus intact; cycle 3
weeks on then one week off in patients with intact uterus)
anastrozole [Arimidex] (Tab 1 mg) 1 mg PO QD
Cenestin [synthetic conjugated estrogens, A] (Tab 0.625, 0.9 mg)) PO 0.625-1.25 mg PO QD✱ *menopause* ★

Climara [estradiol transdermal] (patch 0.05, 0.1 mg/24h) initially one 0.1 mg/24h patch a week, 4 per box•

CombiPatch [estradiol/norethindrone acetate] (patch 0.05/0.14, 0.05/0.25 mg/d) apply patch twice a week

Crinone [Progesterone 8%] (vaginal gel 90 mg/applicatorful) Supplemental 90 mg intravaginally QD; replacement 90 mg intravaginally bid. Progesterone deficiency

Danocrine [danazol] (Tab 50, 100, 200 mg) PO 100-400 mg BID

Esclim [estradiol transdermal] (0.025, 0.0375, 0.05, 0.075, 0.1 mg/24 hours) apply patch twice a week•

Estrace [estradiol] (Tab 0.5, 1, 2 mg) PO 1-2 tabs QD, 3 weeks on, 1 week off•

Estrace Vaginal cream [estradiol] 0.01% cream (42.5g with applicator) 2-4g daily X 1-2 wks, then ½ initial dose daily X 1-2 wks, then 1g 1-3 times/wk

Estraderm [estradiol transdermal] (patch 0.05, 0.1 mg/24h) one patch twice weekly•

estradiol [Vivelle] (0.0375, 0.05, 0.075, 0.1 mg/d patches) Apply twice weekly•

estradiol cypionate IM 1-5 mg Q 3-4 wk

estradiol valerate IM 10-20 mg Q 4 wk

Estratab [plant based estrogen] (Tab 0.3, 0.625, 1.25 mg) PO 0.3-1.25 mg Q D; has been approved for osteoporosis prevention•

Fempatch [Estradiol] (Patch 0.25 mg/d) Apply 1 patch weekly, after 4-6 weeks may use 2 patches•

letrozole [Femara] (Tab 2.5 mg) 2.5 mg PO QD

Premarin [conjugated estrogen] (Tab 0.3, 0.625, 0.9, 1.25, 2.5 mg) PO 1 tab QD•

Premphase [conjugated estrogen 0.625mg QD for 28days & medroxyprogesterone 5mg on days 15-28] PO 1 Tab QD- 28 days

Prempro [conjugated estrogen/medroxyprogesterone 0.625/5 & 0.625/2.5 mg] PO 1 Tab QD- 28 days

Prometrium [progesterone](Cap 100 mg) see package insert for dosing

tamoxifen [Nolvadex] (Tab 10 mg) PO 10-20 mg BID

testosterone transdermal [Testoderm] (4mg/24h, 6mg/24h) Begin 6mg/24h on scrotum QD, if too small use 4mg

Vagifem [estradiol hemihydrate] (Vag Tab 25 mcg) One tab inserted vaginally twice weekly • ★

THYROID

Euthroid [Thyroid equivalent (mg) {thyroxine (μg)/liothyronine (μg)}] (Tab 30{30/7.5}, 60{60/15}, 120{120/30}, 180{180/45}) PO 30-180mg QD

liothyronine [Cytomel, T3, Triostat IV] (Tab 5, 25, 50 μg) PO 5-100 μg QD. Myxedema coma/precoma IV initial dose 25-50 μg or if patient has known heart disease 10-20 μg

methimazole [Tapazole] (Tab 5, 10 mg) PO initial 15-60 mg, then 5-15 mg/d divided TID.

propylthiouracil [PTU] (Tab 50 mg) PO Initial 300 mg/d, then 100-150 mg/d divided TID.

Thyroid USP [desiccated thyroid] (Tab 15, 30, 60, 90, 120, 180, 240, 300 mg) PO 60-120 mg QD.

thyroxine [Synthroid, Levoxyl] (Tab 25, 50, 75, 88, 100, 112,125,137, 150, 175, 200, 300 μg) PO 50-200 μg QD.

thyroxine [Synthroid IV] (vials 200, 500 μg) Myxedema coma initially 100-400 μg IV, then 50-200 μg daily.

Thyrolar [Thyroid equivalent (mg) {thyroxine (μg)/liothyronine (μg)}] (Tab 15{12.5/3.1}, 30{25/6.25}, 60{50/12.5}, 120{100/25}, 180{150/37.5}) PO 30-120 mg QD.

OSTEOPOROSIS (Mayo Clinic Proceedings, OCT 1997, vol 72, 943-49.)

Indications for measuring bone mineral density (BMD): •All perimenopausal & postmenopausal (estrogen deficient) women trying to decide whether to receive estrogen replacement therapy (ERT) or who cannot take ERT and are willing to try alternative therapies. •Pt's with suspected osteoporosis based on spinal x-rays. •Pt's with primary asymptomatic hyperparathyroidism if established bone loss would lead to surgery. •Follow-up to monitor effects of therapy. (generally ≥2years after initial measurement) •BMD should only be measured if results would influence therapy.

WHO Diagnostic Criteria for Osteoporosis

Definition	Criteria
Normal	BMD within 1 SD[1] of RM[2] for young adults
Low Bone Mass (osteopenia)	BMD between -1 & -2.5 SD lower than RM for young adults
Osteoporosis	BMD -2.5 or more SD lower than RM for young adults
Severe osteoporosis (established)	Osteoporosis (as defined above) with 1 or more fragility fractures

[1]RM - Reference Mean. [2]SD - Standard Deviation

MISCELLANEOUS

alendronate sodium [Fosamax] (Tab 5,10, 40 mg) *Osteoporosis prevention* 5 mg QD, *Osteoporosis* 10 mg QD; *Paget's disease of bone* 40 mg QD; take 30 min before first food, beverage, or med of the day. Take with a full glass of water (6-8 oz)

becaplermin [Regranex] (gel 0.01%) ≥16 yrs apply once daily until complete healing occurs. *Diabetic ulcers*

betaine anhydrous [Cystadane](Powder 1g/1.7ml) 3 g PO BID; mix with 4-6oz water until dissolved *Homocystinuria*

46 ENDOCRINOLOGY

<u>bromocriptine</u> [Parlodel] (Tab 2.5 mg; Cap 5 mg) Initially 1.25 mg BID with meals, increase 2.5 mg/day q2-4 weeks to 10-40 mg/d

<u>calcitonin</u> [Calcimar, Miacalcin] (200 IU/ml in 2ml vials, 200IU/spray in 2ml bottle - 14 sprays) SC/IM *Paget's & Postmenopausal osteoporosis* 100 IU/D; *hypercalcemia* 4 IU/kg q12h; NS *Postmenopausal osteoporosis* 200IU intranasally daily, alternate nostrils. MAX 8IU/kg q6h.

<u>desmopressin</u> [DDAVP,] (Scored Tabs 0.1, 0.2 mg; NS 10mcg/spray; Nasal pipets 0.1 mg/ml; Inj 4mcg/ml) *Diabetes insipidus* : Adult intranasal 0.1-0.4ml in single or 2-3 divided doses, Peds 3mo-12yoa 0.05-0.3ml daily; IV/SC 0.5-0.1ml daily in 2 divided doses; *Nocturnal enuresis* ≥6yoa use 1 spray each nostril q HS.

<u>etidronate disodium</u> [Didronel] (Tab 200,400mg)PO *Paget's* 5-10mg/kg/d on an empty stomach 2h before meals

<u>finasteride</u> [Propecia] (Tab 1 mg) PO 1 mg daily

<u>leuprolide</u> [Lupron] (Inj 5 mg/ml) *Initially* 50mcg/kg/day (min 7.5 mg) SC single dose; [Lupron Depot] (Inj 3.75, 7.5 mg/vial), [Lupron Depot-ped] (Inj 7.5, 11.25, 15 mg/kit) 0.3 mg/kg q4 wks as single IM inj. May increase 3.75 mg q4 wks. *Precocious puberty*

<u>pamidronate disodium</u> [Aredia] *Hypercalcemia* IV infusion 60-90 mg over 24h

<u>paricalcitol</u> [Zemplar] Vit D for treatment and prevention of secondary hyperparathyroidism with chronic renal failure

<u>pergolide</u> [Permax] (Tab 0.05, 0.25, 1 mg) Initially, 0.05 mg QD X 2days, then increase 0.1-0.15 mg/day every 3rd day to a mean therapeutic dose of 3 mg/day usually divided TID

<u>raloxifene</u> [Evista] (Tab 60 mg) 60 mg Q D- SERM (selective estrogen receptor modulator) Osteoporosis

<u>risedronate</u> [Actonel] (Tab 30 mg) Paget's - 30 mg once daily for 2 months

<u>sacrosidase</u> [Sucraid] (Sol 8500 I.U./ml; 118 ml bottles) replacement therapy of the genetically determined sucrase deficiency; <= 15 kg: 1 ml/meal or snack (1 scoop or 22 drops); > 15 kg: 2 ml dilute with 2-4 ounces of water, milk or infant formula. Give 1/2 dose before and 1/2 dose after meal

<u>sevelamer</u> [Renagel] (Cap 403mg) 2 to 4 capsules with each meal. *hyperphosphatemia* Category C ★

<u>somatropin</u> [Saizen] (Inj 5 mg/vial) Individualize dose, usually 0.06 mg/kg SC or IM 3 times weekly.

<u>tiludronate</u> [Skelid] (Tab 200 mg) 400 mg PO QD X 3 months. Take with 6-8 ozs water at least 2° before any food, beverage, or medication. *Pagets disease of bone*

Endocrinology Notes:

ANTIHISTAMINES

astemizole [Hismanal] (10 mg tab) 10 mg QD

azatadine maleate [Optimine] (1 mg tab) 1-2 mg BID

azelastine [Astelin] (spray 137 mcg/actuation) ≥ *12 years of age* 2 sprays per nostril BID

brompheniramine maleate [Dimetane] (4, 8, 12 mg tab; 8, 12 mg time release tab; 2 mg/5cc elixir; 10 mg/ml injectable) 4 mg q4-6h, OR, 8-12 mg SR tab q8-12h; 5-20 mg IV/IM/SC

carbinoxamine maleate [Clistin] (4 mg tab) 4-8 mg TID-QID

cetirizine [Zyrtec] (Tabs 5, 10 mg; Syrup 1 mg/ml) *2-5 yoa* ½ tsp QD (Max 5mg QD); *≥6yoa* 5-10 mg QD

chlorpheniramine maleate [Chlor-Trimeton] (2, 4, 8, 12 mg tabs; 8, 12 mg time release tab & capsule; 2 mg/5cc syrup; 10, 100 mg/ml injectable) 4 mg q4-6h, OR, 8-12 mg SR tab q8-12h; 5-20 mg IV/IM/SC

clemastine fumarate [Tavist](1.34,2.68 mg tab; 0.67 mg/5cc syrup) 1.34-2.68 mg TID; *PEDS use* 0.2-0.4 mg/kg/d

cyproheptadine HCl [Periactin] (4 mg tab; 2 mg/5cc syrup) 4-20 mg QD divided TID; *PEDS use* 0.25 mg/kg/d

dexchlorpheniramine maleate [Poladex] (2 mg tab; 4, 6 mg timed release tab; 2 mg/5cc syrup) 2 mg q4-6h, or, 4-6 mg SR tab q8-10h

diphenhydramine [Benadryl] (25, 50 mg tab & capsule; 12.5 mg/5cc elixir & syrup; 10 mg/ml, 50 mg/ml injectable) 25-50 mg PO q6-8h; 10-100 mg IV or deep IM (max 400 mg/day)

fexofenadine [Allegra] Cap 60 mg BID; no differences in adverse events or Qtc interval when administered alone or in combination with erythromycin or ketoconazole.

loratadine [Claritin (Tab/Reditabs 10 mg; Syr 1 mg/ml), Claritin-D (loratadine 5 mg + pseudoephedrine 120 mg), Claritin-D 24° (loratadine 10 mg + pseudoephedrine 240 mg)] *(>6yrs)* 10 mg QD; Claritin-D BID; Claritin-D 24° 1 QD

methdilazine HCl [Tacaryl] (4 mg chewable; 8 mg tab; 4 mg/5cc syrup) 8 mg BID-QID; *PEDS use* 4 mg BID-QID.

phenindamine tartrate [Nolahist] (25 mg tab) 25 mg q4-6h

Poly-Histine (4 mg pheniramine/4 mg pyrilamine/4 mg phenyltoloxamine per 5cc) 10cc q4h; *PEDS (6-12yrs) use* 5cc q4h; *(2-6yrs) use* 2.5cc q4h

promethazine [Phenergan] (12.5, 25, 50 mg tabs & supp; 6.25, 25 mg/5cc syrup; 25, 50 mg/ml injectable) 12.5-50 mg PO/PR/IM/IV q4-6h; *PEDS use* 1 mg/kg

pyrilamine maleate [Nisaval] (25 mg tab) 25-50 mg TID-QID

terfenadine [Seldane (60 mg), Seldane-D discontinued by manufacturer Feb 1, 1998

trimeprazine [Temaril] (2.5 mg tab; 5 mg SR tab; 2.5 mg/5cc syrup) 2.5 mg QID, OR, 5 mg SR tab q12h; *PEDS use* 1.25-2.5 mg TID

tripelennamine HCl [PBZ, PBZ-SR] (25,50 mg tab; 100 mg SR tab; 37.5 mg/5cc elixir) 25-50 mg q4-6h, or, 100 mg SR tab q12h; *PEDS use* 5 mg/kg/day divided in 4-6 doses (max 300 mg/day)

triprolidine HCl [Actidil] (2.5 mg tab; 1.25 mg/5cc syrup) 2.5 mg q4-6h; *PEDS use* 1.25 mg q4-6h

NARCOTIC ANTITUSSIVE COMBINATIONS

Actifed with codeine syrup C5 (1.25 mg triprolidine + 30 mg pseudoephedrine + 10 mg codeine/5cc) 10cc q4-6h; *PEDS (6-12 yrs) use* 5cc; *(2-6 yrs) use* 2.5cc

Brontex C5(10 mg codeine + 300 mg guaifenesin) PO tab: *(>12 yrs)* one tab q4h; liquid *(6-12 yrs)* 10 ml q4h, *(>12 yoa)* 20 ml q4h

Calcidrine C5 (8.4 mg codeine + 152 mg Ca^{2+}-iodide/5cc)10cc q4h; *PEDS (6-10yrs) use* 5cc; *(2-6yrs) use* 2.5cc

Entuss-D C3 (Tab/{Jr liq per 5cc} 5/{2.5} mg hydrocodone+300/{100} mg guaifenesin+30/{30} mg pseudoephedrine) *PEDS liq (6-12yrs) use* 10cc q4-6h, MAX 40cc/24h, Adult Tab 1-1.5 QID

Hycodan C3 (1.5 mg homatropine + 5 mg hydrocodone/5cc) 5cc QID

Phenergan with Codeine C5 (6.25 mg promethazine + 10 mg codeine/5cc syrup) 5cc q4-6h; *PEDS (6-12 yrs) use* 2.5cc; *(2-6 yrs) use* 1.25cc

Robitussin A-C C5 (100 mg guaifenesin + 10 mg codeine/5cc) 10cc q4h; *PEDS (6-12yrs) use* 5cc

Tussionex C3 (10 mg hydrocodone + 8 mg chlorpheniramine/5cc) 5cc q12h; *PEDS (6-12yrs) use* 2.5cc

NON-NARCOTIC ANTITUSSIVE- PURE & COMBINATIONS

benzonatate ℞ [Tessalon Perles] (100 mg capsule) 100 mg TID, max 600 mg/24h

dextromethorphan HBr OTC [various manuf.] (2.5, 5, 7.5 mg lozenges; 3.5, 7.5, 15 mg/5cc liquid; 5, 10 mg/5cc syrup) 10-30 mg q4-8h, max 120 mg/24h; *PEDS (6-12yrs)* use 5-10 mg q4-8h, max 60 mg/24h; *(2-6yrs)* use 2.5-7.5 mg q4-8h, max 30 mg/24h

dextromethorphan HBr/benzocaine OTC [various manuf.] (10 mg/10mg, 5 mg/1.25 mg, 2.5 mg/1 mg lozenges)

diphenhydramine HCl [Benylin Cough] (12.5 mg/5cc syrup) 25 mg q4h, max 150 mg/24h; PEDS *(6-12yrs)* use 12.5 mg, max 75 mg/24h; *(2-6yrs)* use 6.25 mg, max 25 mg/24h

DECONGESTANT/ANTIHISTAMINE COMBINATIONS

Actifed OTC (60 mg pseudoephedrine + 2.5 mg triprolidine/10cc syrup or tab) PO 1 q4-6h, Max 4 tabs in 24h

Contac OTC [phenylpropanolamine/chlorpheniramine] (75 mg/8 mg, 75 mg/12 mg capsule) 1 PO BID

Deconamine ℞ (60 mg pseudoephedrine + 4 mg chlorpheniramine tab) 1 tab TID-QID

Entex [45 mg phenylpropanolamine/5 mg phenylephrine/200 mg guaifenesin TABS] 1 tab PO QID; [20 mg phenylpropanolamine/5 mg phenylephrine/100 mg guaifenesin per 5cc liquid] 10cc PO QID;

Entex LA [75 mg phenylpropanolamine/400 mg guaifenesin TABS] 1 tab PO q2h

Naldecon [40 mg phenylpropanolamine/10 mg phenylephrine/5 mg chlorpheniramine/12 mg phenyltoloxamine TABS] 1 tab TID; [5 mg phenylpropanolamine/1.25 mg phenylephrine/0.5 mg chlorpheniramine/2 mg phenyltoloxamine/5cc] *(6-12yrs)* 10cc q3-4h; *(1-6yrs)* 5cc q3-4h; *(6-12mos)* 2.5cc q3-4h

Ornade Spansules (75 mg phenylpropanolamine + 12 mg chlorpheniramine maleate capsule) 1 tab q12h

Tavist-D (75 mg phenylpropanolamine + 1.34 mg clemastine fumarate tab) 1 tab q12h

Trinalin Repetabs Ŗ (120 mg pseudoephedrine sulfate + 1 mg azatadine maleate tab) 1 tab BID

Phenergan-D Ŗ (60 mg pseudoephedrine + 6.25 mg promethazine tab) 1 tab QID

Phenergan-VC C5 (5 mg phenylephrine + 6.25 mg promethazine/5cc liquid) 5cc q4-6h; PEDS *(6-12yrs)* use 2.5cc; *(2-6yrs)* use 1.25cc

EXPECTORANTS

guaifenesin OTC [Robitussin] (100, 200 mg/5cc liquid; 200 mg capsule; 100, 200 mg tab) 100-400 mg q4h, Max 2.4 g/24h; PEDS *(6-12yrs)* use 100-200 mg, max 1.2 g/24h; *(2-6yrs)* use 50-100 mg, max 600 mg/24h [Humibid LA, Humibid sprinkles] (300 mg SR capsule; 600 mg SR tab) 300-600 mg q12h

terpin hydrate OTC (85 mg/5cc elixir) 85-170 mg TID-QID

INTRANASAL STEROIDS

beclomethasone [Vancenase AQ, Vancenase AQ Double Strength] (42 mcg/spray; DS 84 mcg/spray) 42mcg each nostril BID-QID; OR 84 mcg each nostril QD-BID

beclomethasone dipropionate [Beconase, Vancenase] (16.8 g canister; 25 g bottle) 1 inhal each nostril BID-QID

budesonide [Rhinocort] (32mcg/actuation) 2 sprays each nostril BID or 4 sprays each nostril QD

dexamethasone sodium phosphate [Decadron Phosphate Turbinaire](12.6g bottle) 2 sprays (168µg) BID-TID

flunisolide [Nasalide] (25cc bottle) 2 sprays (50 mcg) each nostril BID

fluticasone propionate [Flonase] (0.05%) 2 sprays (200 mcg) each nostril QD

mometasone fumarate [Nasonex] (50 mcg/spray) >12 yoa 2 sprays each nostril BID

triamcinolone acetonide [Nasacort] (15 g container) 2 sprays (110 mcg) each nostril QD

NASAL DECONGESTANTS

epinephrine OTC [Adrenalin Chloride] (0.1% in 30cc container) Apply locally

ephedrine OTC (0.25% spray; 0.5% drops; 1% jelly) Product specific dosing - see label

naphazoline HCl [Privine] (0.05% sol 25cc drops; 20cc or 473cc spray)1-2 sprays or drops each nostril q6h

oxymetazoline HCl (0.025% in 20cc drops; 0.05% in drops & spray) 2-3 sprays or drops each nostril TID

phenylpropanolamine OTC (25, 50 mg tabs, 75 mg capsule time-released) 25 mg q4h, OR, 75 mg SR q12h

pseudoephedrine sulfate OTC (120 mg extended release tab) 1 tab q12h

pseudoephedrine HCl OTC [Sudafed] (30, 60 mg tab; 120 mg ext. release; 15, 30 mg/15ml liquid; 7.5 mg/0.8cc drops) ADULTS use 60 mg q4-6h, OR, 120 mg q12h

phenylephrine HCl OTC [Neo-Synephrine] (0.125%, 0.16%, 0.25%, 0.5%, 1% solution) 2-3 sprays or drops in each nostril q3-4h prn

tetrahydrozoline HCl [Tyzine] (0.05%, 0.1% solution in 15cc, 30cc drops, & 15cc spray) 2-4 drops or sprays each nostril q4h

xylometazoline HCl [Otrivin] (0.05%, 0.1% solution in 25cc drops, & 20cc spray) 2-3 drops or sprays q8-10h

OTIC PREPARATIONS

Auralgan Otic [1.4% benzocaine/5.4% antipyrine in 10 ml sol] 2-4 drops, insert cotton pledget, TID/QID

Americaine Otic [20% benzocaine/0.1% benzethonium chloride in 15 ml] 4-5 drops, insert cotton pledget, q1-2h

Cerumenex Drops Ŗ [10% triethanolamine polypeptide in 6 & 12 ml] Fill ear, insert cotton, flush in 15-30 min

Chloromycetin Otic [0.5% chloramphenicol in 15 ml with dropper] 2-3 drops TID

Cortisporin Otic [1% hydrocortisone/5 mg/ml neomycin/10,000u polymyxin B 10 ml sol or susp] 4 drops TID/QID

Cortisporin-TC Otic [Colistin sulfate, Neomycin, hydrocortisone, thonzonium, polysorbate] (Susp 10 mL) Adults 4 drops in affected ear TID-QID; PEDS 3 drops TID-QID

Debrox Otic [6.5% carbamide peroxide in 30 ml] 5-10 drops BID up to 4 days

ofloxacin [Floxin Otic](Sol 0.3%, 5 ml) 1-12 yoa 5 drops BID x 10 D, >12 yoa 10 drops BID x 10 D

MISCELLANEOUS

cromolyn sodium OTC [Nasalcrom] (13, 26cc metered spray device) 1 spray each nostril 3-6 times daily

ipratropium bromide [Atrovent Nasal Spray] (0.03%= 42 mcg, 0.06%=84 mcg) 0.03% 2 sprays/nostril 2-3 times/d -approved for symptomatic relief of allergic and non-allergic perennial rhinitis; 0.06% 2 sprays/nostril 3-4 times/d

scopolamine (Transderm Scop) [Patch 1.5mg] apply q3 days prn to prevent motion sickness

FLUID MANAGEMENT OBJECTIVES
- Beware of treating a lab value! Lab values may be erroneous from sampling, labeling, or running the sample.
- Always correlate the patient's condition with lab values.
- Treat abnormalities at approximately the rate at which they developed. As a general rule, correct half the deficit, then reassess and correct the remaining deficit gradually.
- Multiple fluid, electrolyte, & acid/base abnormalities should be corrected in the following sequence: 1st Fluid volume & perfusion deficits; 2nd pH; 3rd K^+, Ca^{2+}, & Mg^{2+} abnormalities; 4th Na^+ & Cl^- abnormalities.
- NOTE: When fluid & perfusion deficits are corrected, many pH & elect. abnormalities will correct themselves.
- Remember that acidosis is often associated with ↑K^+, ↑Ca^{2+}, & ↑Mg^{++}. Alkalosis lowers K^+, Ca^{2+}, & Mg^{++}. If hypokalemia occurs with severe acidosis, then suspect lab error or severe hypokalemia.
- Generally, if all electrolytes are equally low, then symptoms will be less severe than if only one is low.

MAINTENANCE REQUIREMENTS
(Guidelines only - actual requirements may vary considerably depending on patient's specific condition.)
- 70kg male: D5½NS with 20 mEq KCl/liter at 125ml/hr, (≈3 liters of free water.)
- Other adults & pediatrics: D5½NS with 20 mEq KCl/liter, use formula below to determine rate.
- NOTE: The above guidelines are based on the usual fluid requirement necessary to maintain a urine output of ≈1-1.5 L/24h. Urine output & daily weights are useful in monitoring fluid & perfusion status.
- NOTE: Ca^{2+}, Mg^{2+}, PO_4^-, protein, & vitamins may be necessary after 5-7 days of IV fluids.

ABNORMAL LOSS GUIDELINES
- Insensible losses ↑ 100-150 ml/24h for each degree >37°C. Replace insensible losses with D5W. Sweat is a sensible loss; replace with NS.
- Third space losses should be replaced with NS or LR.
- Other losses should be guided by frequent monitoring of pts. clinical status.

COMMONLY USED FORMULAS IN IV FLUID THERAPY
- Serum osmolarity = 2(Na+) + [glucose/18] + BUN/2.8)
- Effective Osmols = 2(Na+) + [glucose/18] + mannitol (mosm) + sorbitol + glycerol
  {effective osmols are those solutes which do not cross easily into muscle cells}
- Colloidal osmotic pressure = 5.5(albumin) + 1.4(globulin)
- Desired TBW = [measured serum Na+ x current TBW] / normal serum Na+
- Body water deficit = desired TBW − current TBW
- Water deficit (L) = current TBW x [(measured serum Na+/normal serum Na+) − 1]
- Serum Na+ correction for hyperglycemia = [((observed gluc − normal gluc) x1.4) / normal gluc] + observed Na+

BASICS	DAILY ELECTROLYTE REQUIREMENTS

TBW = 60% of body weight (BW)
• Intracellular is 40% of BW,
• Extracellular is 20% of BW,
  Plasma is 5% of BW,
  Interstitial is 15% of BW.
Water Balance
Intake ≈ 2500 ml/24h (≈35ml/kg/24h)
• oral liquids ≈ 1,500ml/24h
• oral solids ≈ 700ml/24h
• metabolic ≈ 250ml/24h
Output ≈ 1400-2300ml/24h
• urine ≈ 800-1500ml/24h
• stool ≈ 250ml/24h
• insensible (skin & lungs) ≈600-900ml/24h
	Na+(as NaCl) = 80-120 mEq/24h
	 (Peds = 3-4mEq/kg/24h)
	Cl- (as NaCl) = 80-120 mEq/24h
	K+ = 50-100 mEq/24h;
	 (Peds = 2-3 mEq/kg/24h)
	NOTE: K+ is mostly excreted in urine if not
	hypokalemic or with normal renal function. Also,
	note[K+] changes with changes in pH.
	Ca2+ = 1-3 gm/24h*;Mg2+ = 20 mEq/24h
	 (not routinely needed without indications)
	Glucose = 100-200gm/24h;
	 (Peds = 100-200mg/kg/24h)
	NOTE: Protein sparing: 1 gm glucose/24h
	decreases protein loss by 1/2

BASELINE FLUID REQUIREMENTS	
(First 10kg BW = 100ml/kg/24h) + (Second 10kg BW = 50ml/kg/24h) + (Weight >20kg = 20ml/kg/24h) (70kg Adult = 35ml/kg/24h)	

ELECTROLYTE CONCENTRATION IN BODY FLUIDS (mEq/L)

Fluid	Na⁺	K⁺	Cl⁻	HCO₃⁻	Vol/24*
Saliva	20-60	10-20	15-30	30-50	1-2L
Bile	130-145	4-6	95-105	20-40	0.1-1L
Stomach	40-100	5-15	15-20	0	1.5-2.5L
Pancreas	130-140	4-6	40-75	80-115	1-2L
Sm. Bowel	130-140	4-6	40-60	80-100	1-3L
Colon	80-140	25-45	80-100	30-50	.1-.6L
Diarrhea	50-60	40-50	35-45	45-60	variable
Sweat	40-50	5-10	40-60	0	.2-1.5L

FREQUENTLY USED IV FLUIDS (mEq/L)

Fluid	Glucose	Na⁺	K⁺	Cl⁻	HCO₃⁻	mosm/L	Kcal/L
D5W	50g	0	0	0	0	252	170
D10W	100g	0	0	0	0	505	340
D50W	500g	0	0	0	0	2520	1700
1/2NS (0.45%NS)	0	77	0	77	0	154	0
NS (0.9%NS)	0	154	0	154	0	308	0
3% NS	0	513	0	513	0	1026	0
D5¼NS	50g	38	0	38	0	329	170
D5½NS	50g	77	0	77	0	406	170
D5NS	50g	154	0	154	0	560	170
LR	0	130	4	110	27*	272	<10
D5LR	50g	130	4	110	27*	524	180
Albumin	0	145	0	145	0	unk	unk

*HCO₃⁻ is produced by the liver from lactate

Fluid Notes:

H. Pylori

H. Pylori Treatment Regimens

- omeprazole (Prilosec) 20 mg BID, clarithromycin (Biaxin) 500 mg BID, amoxicillin 1 gm BID or metronidazole 250 mg QID for 14 days (91%[†]) [$290]
- metronidazole 250 mg QID, Pepto-Bismol 525 mg QID, amoxicillin 500 mg QID or tetracycline 500 mg QID for 14 days, H₂RA BID for 28 days (89%[†]) [$190]
- lansoprazole (Prevacid) 30 mg BID, clarithromycin 500mg BID, amoxicillin 1 gm BID for 14 days (96%[†]) [$240]
- omeprazole 40mg Q AM, clarithromycin 500 mg TID for 14 days; then omeprazole 20 mg QD for 14 days (86%[†])[$300]
- omeprazole 40 mg Q AM, metronidazole 250 mg TID, Pepto-Bismol 525 mg QID, amoxicillin 500 mg BID or tetracycline 500 mg QID for 10 days (85%[†])[$140]
- omeprazole 20mg QID, clarithromycin 500mg BID, metronidazole 250mg bid for 7 days (84%[†]) [$140]
- metronidazole 250 mg TID, Pepto-Bismol 525 mg QID, amoxicillin 500 mg BID or tetracycline 500 mg QID for 14 days (80-90%[†]) [$20]
- omeprazole 40 mg Q AM, metronidazole 250 mg TID, amoxicillin 500 mg BID or tetracycline 500 mg QID for 7 days (76%[†]) [$105]

[≈Cost per course], [†] eradication rates; *Am J of Gastroenterol* 1997 Apr;92(4 Suppl):30-34S

PROGNOSTIC SIGNS of ACUTE PANCREATITIS (Ranson's Criteria)

AT ADMISSION OR DIAGNOSIS			DURING INITIAL 48 HS		
Parameter	Non-gallstone	Gallstone	Parameter	Non-gallstone	Gallstone
Age	>55	>70	Hct decrease	>10	>10
WBC	>16,000/m³	>18,000/m³	BUN rise	>5 mg%	>2 mg%
Serum glucose	>200 mg%	>220 mg%	Serum Ca²⁺§	<8 mg%	<8 mg%
LDH	>350 IU/L	>400 IU/L	PaO₂	<60 mmHg	
AST (SGOT)	>250 IU/dL	>250 U/dL	Base deficit	>4 mEq/L	>5 meq/L
			Fluid deficit	>6 L	>4 L
≤2 items ≈5% mortality 3-4 Items ≈15-20% mortality 5-6 items ≈40% mortality ≥ 7 items approach 100% mortality §*Serum Ca²⁺ <7 mg% associated with more serious prognosis*					

ENDOSCOPIC CLASSIFICATION OF GERD SEVERITY

<u>Grade 0</u>: No observed abnormalities in esophageal mucosa

<u>Grade 1</u>: Erythema or diffusely red esophageal mucosa with modest edema that accentuates mucosal folds.

<u>Grade 2</u>: Isolated, round, or linear superficial ulcerations or erosions involving < 10% of the last 5 cm of the esophageal squamous mucosal surface; does not involve the entire esophageal circumference

<u>Grade 3</u>: Extensive superficial ulcerations or erosion involving > 10% to 50% of the last 5 cm of the esophageal squamous mucosal surface; lesions extend around the entire circumference of the esophagus; stenosis not apparent

<u>Grade 4</u>: Deep ulceration anywhere in the esophagus; confluent erosion involving > 50% of the last 5 cm of the esophageal squamous mucosal surface; esophageal stenosis (stricturing) may be present; columnar epithelium found in esophageal lining

VIRAL HEPATITIS

<u>Hepatitis A</u>: •Fecal-oral route, raw shellfish ingestion; •15-50days incubation; •excellent prognosis; •no chronic liver disease; •IgM α-HAV(+) is diagnostic for acute illness, persists for 2-6mos; •IgG α-HAV indefinitely post infection and confers lifetime immunity •children often subclinical or non-icteric; •Immune serum globulin for household contacts.•Vaccine is now available (RNA virus)

<u>Hepatitis B</u>:

- *Transmission*: parenteral, mucous membrane contact of body fluids (eg, blood, saliva), sexual contact, or fetal-maternal; HBV can maintain infectivity on environmental surfaces; •Most adult infections are subclinical; • Diagnosis of acute infection with HBsAg (infrequently absent) OR IgM Anti-HBc (always ↑ with onset of clinical hepatitis); •HBsAg & HBeAg ↑ 1-12 wks after exposure; •clinical hepatitis follows HBsAg by 1-7 wks; •HBsAg & HBeAg levels undetectable several wks after clinical hepatitis resolved unless chronic carrier state; •HBeAg(+) >10wks usually indicates persistent infection; •HBeAg(+) & HBV-DNA indicate replicative phase & are markers for patients likely to transmit infection; •HBsAg(+) and anti-HBe(+) patients are less likely to transmit infection then HBsAg(+) and HBeAg(+) patients; •Anti-HBs usually appears after HBsAg disappears from blood; Anti-HBs that appears during antigenemia and before clinical hepatitis has been associated with arthritis & rash associated with immune complex formation. (DNA virus)

Serologic Markers for Hepatitis B						Anti-HBc	
Infection Stage	LFT[y]	HBsAg	Anti-HBs	HBeAg	Anti-HBe	IgG	IgM
Recent hepatitis B vaccination	N	–	++	–	–	–	–
Hepatitis B late incubation period	↑	+	–	+/–	–	–	–
Acute hepatitis B	↑↑	+	–	+	–	+	+
Acute hepatitis B HBsAg-negative	↑↑	–	+/–[z]	–	–	+	+
Healthy HBsAg carrier	N	+	–	–	+	+++	+/–
Chronic hepatitis B, high infectivity	↑/N	+	–	+	–	+++	+/–
Chronic hepatitis B, low infectivity	↑/N	+	–	–	+	+++	+/–
Hepatitis B infection, recent past	N	–	++	–	+	++	+/–
Hepatitis B infection, distant past	N	–	+/–	–	–	+/–	–

[y]Liver Function Tests   [z]↑ 4-12 wks after exposure

Hepatitis C: •MC cause of post-transfusion hepatitis; •Risk factors - blood transfusions, IV drug abuse, needle sticks, sexual; •Usually presents with chronic, asymptomatic elevation of transaminases which characteristically fluctuate; •50-60% of "cryptogenic" cirrhosis is due to HCV; •Chronic infection in 50%; cirrhosis in 20%; •HCV Pts with cirrhosis have increased risk of hepatocellular CA & are less likely to respond to interferon-α; •Chronic HCV infection may be associated with cryoglobulinemia; Interferon-α normalizes transaminase levels in 40-50% of Pts. (Double stranded RNA virus)

Hepatitis D: •Delta agent requires HBsAg to cause infection; •HDV is strongly associated with IV drug abuse;•Dx with α-HDV seroconversion; •Duration of infection determined by duration of Hep B infection; •May markedly ↑ severity of chronic hepatitis B; •May occur in liver transplants. (defective RNA particle)

Hepatitis E: •Enterically transmitted & clinically resembles hepatitis A; •May be fulminant if acquired during third trimester; •No chronic HEV infection reported. (RNA virus)

Autoimmune hepatitis: •mainly occurs in 10-20yr old female, usually with an insidious onset; •Must rule out Hx of drug-related hepatitis, HBV, HCV, or Wilson's disease; •ANA, smooth muscle antibodies, soluble liver antigen antibodies, & antibodies to liver/kidney microsomal (LKM) antigens are often present; •Hashimoto's thyroiditis, Coombs' positive hemolytic anemia, DM, glomerulonephritis are associated conditions; •Marked ↑'s in serum γ-globulin is common; •60-80% improve with corticosteroids; •Changes in LFT's & γ -globulins are often dramatic; Relapse often occurs, so maintenance therapy is often required
*Principles and Practices of Infectious Diseases, Mandel, Douglas, & Bennett, 4th edition, 1995
Harrison's Principles of Internal Medicine, Fauci et. al., 14th edition, 1998

DIARRHEA MEDICATIONS

attapulgite [Kaopectate] (Susp) 30cc PO after loose stool, 6-12yo use 5cc, 3-6yo use 7.5cc
bismuth subsalicylate [Pepto-Bismol] (Susp 262, 524mg/15cc; Tab 262mg) 2 tabs or 30cc PO q 1h, MAX 8 doses/24h
Donnagel OTC [kaolin 6g/pectin 142.8mg/hyoscyamine 0.1mg/atropine 0.02mg/scopolamine 6.5 mcg per 30cc] (Susp) 30cc PO first dose, then 15cc PO q 3hr prn
furazolidone [Furoxone] (Tab 100 mg, Liq 50 mg/15cc) Adults: 60cc or 1 tab QID; PEDS: 1 month to 1 yo use 2.5-5cc QID, 1 to 4 yo use 5-7.5cc QID, >5 yo use 7.5-15cc QID
Lomotil [Tab diphenoxylate 2.5mg/atropine 0.025mg & per 5cc] 10cc or 2 tabs PO QID
loperamide [Imodium] (Liq 1mg/5cc, Caplets 2mg) Adults: 4mg PO, repeat 2mg prn up to 16mg/24h; PEDS 13-20kg use 1mg TID, 20-30kg use 2mg BID, >30 kg use 2mg TID
Motofen [difenoxin 1mg/atropine 0.025mg] (Tab) 2 tabs PO first, then 1 tab q 3-4h prn
octreotide acetate [Sandostatin] (Amps with 50 mcg/ml, 100 mcg/ml, 500 mcg/ml) Begin with 50 mcg SC/IV q 8h X 48h, if no response, may increase gradually to 500 mcg q 8h

NAUSEA MEDICATIONS

benzquinamide HCl [Emete-Con] (Vials 50mg) 50mg IM q 3-4h; 25mg SIVP(0.5-1cc/min) single dose then IM inj
buclizine HCl [Bucladin-S Softab] (Tab 50mg) 1 tab dissolved in mouth TID prn nausea
chlorpromazine [Thorazine] (Tab 10, 25, 50mg; Supp 25, 100mg; Vials 25mg/cc) 10-25mg PO/IM q 6h prn ; 100mg supp q 6-8h prn

cyclizine [Marezine] (Tab 50mg) *Adults* 50mg ⅓ h prior to departure, repeat q 4-6; *Peds (6-12yrs)* 25mg PRN up to TID. (MAX 200mg/day)

dimenhydrinate [Dramamine] (Tab 50mg) 1 tab PO/IM/IV q 4h

diphenhydramine [Benadryl] (Cap 25, 50mg; Inj 10, 50mg/cc) *ADULTS:* 25-50mg PO/IM/IV TID/QID. *PEDS:* 12.5-25mg PO TID/QID (5mg/kg/24h injectable)

dolasetron [Anzemet] (Tab 50, 100 mg; Inj 20 mg/ml) *Chemotherapy-induced nausea: Adults* use 1.8 mg/kg IV OR 100 mg PO. *Peds 2-16yoa* use 1.8 mg/kg IV/PO. *Postoperative nausea: Adults* use 12.5 mg IV OR 100 mg PO; *Peds 2-16yoa* use 0.35 mg/kg IV OR 1.2 mg/kg PO. IV doses given ≈15-30 min before chemo or before end of surgery; PO doses given within 1-2 hours before chemo or surgery. MAX 100 mg/dose

dronabinol [Marinol]C2(Cap 2.5,5,10mg) 5mg/m² 1-3h before chemo, then q2-4h (4-6 times/day) MAX 15mg/m²

droperidol [Inapsine] (2.5 mg/cc) 1.25-2.5 mg IV/IM

granisetron [Kytril] (Inj 1 mg/ml; Tab 1 mg) IV 10 mcg/kg over 5min, give 30min before chemo (dilute in 20-50ml), *Oral* 1 mg up to 1 hour before chemotherapy and 1 mg 12 hours after first dose

meclizine HCl [Antivert, Bonine] (Tab 12.5, 25, 50 mg) 25-50 mg PO q 24h prn nausea

metoclopramide [Reglan] (Tab 5, 10 mg; Syp 5 mg/5cc; Inj 5 mg/cc) 10 mg PO/IM/IV 1h ac & HS

ondansetron [Zofran] (Inj 2 mg/cc; Tab 4, 8 mg; Sol 4 mg/5ml) to prevent nausea with chemotherapy 32 mg IVPB dose over 15 min. OR, three 0.15 mg/kg 4 h apart

perphenazine [Trilafon] (Tab 2, 4, 8, 16 mg; Liq 16 mg/5cc) 8-16 mg PO QD in divided doses

phosphorated carbohydrate solution [Emetrol] (cherry liquid) *ADULTS:* 15-30cc PO prn; *PEDS:* 5-10cc PO prn

prochlorperazine [Compazine] (Tab 5, 10, 25 mg; Syp 5 mg/cc) begin with 5-10 mg PO TID/QID, (Spansule 10. 15, 30 mg) 10-30mg PO q am/q 12h. (Supp 25 mg) 25 mg PR q 12h. (Inj 5 mg/cc) 2.5-10 mg SIVP/IM q 4h

promethazine [Phenergan] (Tab/Supp 12.5, 25, 50 mg; Syp 6.25, 25 mg/cc) 25-50mg PO/PR/IM q 4h

scopolamine (Transderm Scop) [Patch 1.5 mg] apply q3 days prn to prevent motion sickness

thiethylperazine [Torecan] (Tab/Supp 10 mg, Amps 10 mg/2ml) PO/PR/IM 10-30 mg/d in divided doses

trimethobenzamide [Tigan] (Tab 100, 250 mg; Supp 100, 200 mg; Inj 100 mg/cc) *ADULTS* – 250 mg PO TID/QID, 100 mg PR TID/QID; *PEDS <30 lb*- 100 mg PR TID/QID; *30-90 lb*- 100-200 mg PO/PR TID/QID

ANTICHOLINERGICS & ANTISPASMODICS

anisotropine methylbromide [Valpin 50] (50mg TABS) 50mg TID

clidinium bromide [Quarzan] (2.5, 5mg CAPS) 2.5-5mg TID/QID

dicyclomine HCl [Bentyl] (20mg TAB; 10mg CAP; 10mg/5ml syrup; 10mg/ml inj) Begin with 80mg/day PO divided QID, advance to 160mg/day PO divided; OR, 80mg/day IM only divided QID

glycopyrrolate [Robinul] (1, 2mg TABS; 0.2mg/ml inj) 0.1-0.2mg PO/IM/IV TID/QID.

hexocyclium methylsulfate [Tral Filmtabs] (25mg TABS) 25mg PO AC & HS

hyoscyamine [Levsin] (Tab 0.125mg, Elx 0.125mg/5cc, Drop 0.125mg/cc, Inj 0.5mg/cc) ≥*12 yrs* 1-2 tabs or 5-10cc q 4h prn. *2-12 yrs* ½-1 tab or 1.25-5cc Elx or ¼-1cc drop q 4h

≤*2 yrs* use drops according to weight:

Wt.	Dose	Max/24h		Wt.	Dose	Max/24h
2.3kg	3 drops	18 drops		7 kg	6 drops	36 drops
3.4kg	4 drops	24 drops		10 kg	8 drops	48 drops
5 kg	5 drops	30 drops		15 kg	11 drops	66 drops

isopropamide iodide [Darbid] (Tab 5 mg) PO 5-10 mg BID

mepenzolate bromide [Cantil] (Tab 25 mg) PO 25-50 mg AC & HS

methantheline bromide [Banthine] (Tab 50 mg) PO 50-100 mg q 6h

methscopolamine [Pamine] (Tab 2.5 mg) PO 2.5 mg 30 mins before meals, & 2.5-5 mg at HS

oxyphencyclimine HCl [Daricon] (Tab 10mg) PO 5-10 mg BID/TID

propantheline bromide [Pro-Banthine] (Tab 7.5, 15 mg) PO 15mg 30mins before meals & HS; *PEDS (antisecretory):* 1.5mg/kg/day divided TID/QID

tridihexethyl chloride [Pathilon] (Tab 25mg) PO 25-50 mg AC & HS

ANTICHOLINERGIC COMBINATIONS

Bellergal-S [0.2mg alkaloids of belladonna/40mg phenobarbital/0.6mg ergotamine] 2 Tabs PO QD

Donnatal [0.0194mg atropine/0.0065mg scopolamine/0.1037mg hyoscyamine/16.2mg phenobarbital Tab & elix/5cc] PO 3-8 Tabs/Tsp QD

Donnatal #2 [same as Donnatal with 32.4mg phenobarbital] PO 3-6 Tabs QD

Donnatal Extentabs [0.0582mg atropine/0.0195mg scopolamine/0.3111mg hyoscyamine/48.6mg phenobarbital] PO 2-3 Tabs QD

Levsin w/phenobarbital [0.125 hyoscyamine/15mg phenobarbital Tab & elixir/5cc] PO 3-8 Tabs/Tsp QD

Librax [2.5mg clidinium/5mg chlordiazepoxide] PO 3-8 Tabs QD

H₂ RECEPTOR ANTAGONISTS

nizatidine [Axid {Axid AR OTC 75 mg}] (Cap 150, 300 mg) 150 mg BID or 300 mg QD; maintenance - 150 mg q hs; Axid AR 75 mg BID prn

famotidine [Pepcid, Pepcid RPD (orally disintegrating tab), {Pepcid AC OTC Tab and chewable 10 mg}] (Tab 20, 40mg; RPD 20, 40 mg; Susp 40mg/5cc; Vials 10mg/cc) Pepcid 20mg PO BID or 40mg PO QD; 20mg IVP or IVPB q 12h. Pepcid AC 10 mg BID prn

cimetidine [Tagamet, {Tagamet HB OTC 200 mg}] Tab 200, 300, 400, 800mg; Liq 300mg/5cc) Tagamet 300mg PO/IM/IV QID or 800mg PO BID or 400mg PO q hs. GERD—1600mg in divided doses. Continuous IV = 37.5mg/hr. Tagamet HB- 200 mg bid prn

ranitidine [Zantac {Zantac 75 OTC 75 mg}] (Tab 150, 300 mg; EFFERdose Tab & granules 150mg; GELdose 150, 300 mg; Syp 15 mg/cc; Vials 25 mg/cc, 50 mg/50cc premixed) 150 mg PO BID or 300 mg PO q hs. 50 mg SIVP q 6-8h or 6.25 mg/hr continuous IV; Zantac 75 OTC 75 mg BID prn

H⁺/K⁺ ATPase ENZYME INHIBITORS

lansoprazole [Prevacid] (Cap 15, 30mg) *Duodenal ulcer* 15mg QD for 4 wks; *Erosive esophagitis* 30mg QD 8-16 wks; *ZE syndrome initially* 60mg/d; doses up to 90mg BID have been used (give >90mg/d in divided doses)

omeprazole [Prilosec] (20 mg delayed release capsules) *Duodenal ulcer & Erosive esophagitis* 20 mg QD X 4-8 wks; *Gastric ulcer* 40mg QD X 4-8wks *ZE syndrome initially* 60mg/d, doses up to 120mg TID have been used (doses >80mg/day should be divided)

rabeprazole [AcipHex] (Tab 20 mg) *Erosive/Ulcerative esophagitis* 20 mg QD X 4-8 wks, maintenance 20 mg QD; *Duodenal ulcer* 20 mg QD X 4 wks; *Zollinger Ellison Syndrome* initially 60 mg QD, 100mg QD or 60mg BID may be required ★

ANTACIDS & ANTI-GAS PREPARATIONS

aluminum hydroxide [ALternaGEL, Alu-Cap, Amphojel, Dialume] 5cc (600 mg) PO q 4h

aluminum carbonate gel [Basaljel] (Susp & Cap) 10cc or 2 capsules PO q 2h prn

Maalox [aluminum hydroxide, magnesium hydroxide, Maalox plus add simethicone] 15-30cc or 1 tablet PO prn

Mylanta [aluminum hydroxide, magnesium hydroxide, Mylanta II add simethicone] 15-30cc or 1 tablet PO prn

sodium citrate dihydrate [Citra pH] 30cc PO QD prn

simethicone [Mylicon, Mylanta Gas] (Liq 40mg/0.6ml, Chew 40, 80,125mg) PO 40-125mg QID after meals or prn

simethicone + activated charcoal [Flatulex] 1 tablet PO TID prn; [Charcoal Plus] 2 tablets PO QID prn

GI STIMULANTS

cisapride [Propulsid] (Tab 10, 20mg) 10mg PO 15min AC & HS, may ↑ to 20mg QID

dexpanthenol [Ilopan] (250mg/ml in 2ml amps) 250-500mg IM, repeat in 2h, then q 6h; May mix with bulk IV solutions. *Treatment & prevention of adynamic ileus*

Ilopan-Choline [Tabs 50mg dexpanthenol/25mg choline] 2-3 tabs PO TID

metoclopramide [Reglan] (Tab 5, 10mg; Syp 5mg/5cc; Inj 5mg/cc) 10mg PO/IM/IV 1h ac & HS

BULK LAXATIVES

calcium polycarbophil [FiberCon] (Tab 625 mg) 2 - 8 tabs PO q d for 1-3 days

methylcellulose [Citrucel] 1 tbs in 8 oz liquid QD/BID/TID. OTC

psyllium [Metamucil, Fiberall, Mylanta Natural Fiber, Perdiem Fiber] (powder, effervescent powder, wafers) usually 1 tsp, 1 wafer, or 1 packet 1 - 3 times daily. Take with at least 8 oz. of liquid

COMBINATION LAXATIVES

Dialose Plus, Correctol [Tab 100 mg docusate sodium + 65 mg phenolphthalein] 1-2 tablets at HS prn

Haley's M-O [25% mineral oil + Magnesium hydroxide] 15-30cc q HS prn

Perdiem [82% psyllium + 18% senna] 5-10cc in 8 oz liquid q d prn

Peri-Colace [Tab 30mg casanthranol + 100mg docusate sodium; Syp 30mg casanthranol + 60mg docusate per 5cc] 1-2 caps or 15-30cc at HS prn

Senokot-S [Tab 8.6mg sennosides+50mg docusate sodium] ≥12yrs 2 tabs qd;6-12yrs 1 tab qd;2-6yrs ½ tab qd

OSMOTIC LAXATIVES

lactulose [Chronulac] (667 mg/ml) *Constipation* use 15-30ml PO q d prn, can be increased to 60ml q d prn; [Cephulac] *Hepatic encephalopathy* use 30-45ml PO TID/QID

sorbitol 2cc/kg of 70% solution PO q d prn up to 50cc

SALINE LAXATIVES

Fleet enema [Adult, Children's, Mineral Oil] (monobasic & dibasic sodium phosphate) 1 enema QD prn. OTC

Fleet Phospho-Soda (2.4 g monobasic sodium) ≥12 yrs use 20cc QD; 10-12 yrs use 10cc QD; 5-10 yrs use 5cc QD. Mix recommended dose with 4 oz liquid, follow with 8 oz liquid. OTC

STOOL SOFTENERS
docusate sodium [Colace, Dialose] (Tab 50, 100, 250 mg; Liq 20, 50 mg/cc) 100-300 mg daily prn
mineral oil 5-30cc PO q HS prn. OTC

STIMULANT LAXATIVES
Castor Oil *Adults use* 15-30cc PO q HS. *Peds use* 5-15cc PO q HS
Ceo-Two (Supp sodium bicarbonate + potassium bitartrate) 1-2 supp PR q 4-6h prn
Dulcolax (bisacodyl Tab 5mg; Supp 10mg) *≥12yrs* use 2-3 tabs or 1 supp QD; *6-12yrs* 1 tab; *≤12yrs* ½ supp QD
Fleet Babylax (glycerin - 4cc rectal applicators) 2-6 yrs use 1 applicator PR QD prn. OTC
Fleet Bisacodyl enema (10 mg bisacodyl in 30cc) ≥12 yrs use 30cc PR QD; 6-12 yrs use 15cc PR QD. OTC
Fleet Flavored Castor Oil emulsion ≥12 yrs use 45cc PO QD; 2-12 yrs use 15cc PO QD. OTC
Fleet Prep kit Use according to kit instructions
glycerin (Supp) 1 PR prn. OTC
magnesium citrate 4cc/kg PO prn up to 300cc. OTC
magnesium hydroxide (Milk of Magnesia) (Tab 325 mg; Liq 390 mg/5cc) 5-15cc PO prn. OTC
Senokot (Tab 8.6 mg; Granules 15 mg/5cc; SenokotXtra tab 17 mg) ≥12 yrs 2 tabs QD; 6-12 yrs 1 tab QD; 2-6 yrs ½ tab QD

MISCELLANEOUS GI AGENTS
chenodiol [Chenix] (Tab 250 mg) 250-500 mg PO BID
Helidac [bismuth subsalicylate, metronidazole, tetracycline] PO 2 bismuth 262.4mg, 1 metronidazole 250mg, 1 tetracycline 500mg QID for 14 days in combination with H2 antagonist; 82% H. Pylori eradication rate
infliximab [Remicade] (IV 100mg in 20 ml vial) PO 1 mg daily. monoclonal antibody for the treatment of Crohn's disease- moderate-to-severe: 5 mg/kg given as a single IV infusion; fistulizing: Administer an initial 5 mg/kg dose followed with additional 5 mg/kg doses at 2 and 6 weeks after the first infusion
Ku-Zyme (75 mg lipase, 30 mg amylase, 6 mg protease, 2 mg cellulase) 1-2 capsules PO AC
mesalamine [Rowasa, Asacol, Pentasa] (Enema 4 g in 60cc, Supp 500 mg, Tab 400 mg, Pentasa 250 mg caps) 4 g enema q HS; 1 supp PR BID; 2 tabs PO TID; 4 Pentasa caps QID
misoprostol [Cytotec] (100, 200 mcg TABS) 100-200 mcg PO QID with food
olsalazine [Dipentum] (250mg CAPS) 1gm daily in 2 divided doses with food
pancreatin [Creon, Donnazyme, Entozyme] 1-3 tabs PO AC
pancrelipase [Viokase, Pancrease, Cotazym, Ku-Zyme HP, Ultrase, Zymase] (lipase, amylase, protease) 1-3 tabs PO AC
Prevpac (2- lansoprazole 30 mg , 2- clarithromycin 500 mg and 4- amoxicillin 500 mg) PO take lansoprazole 30 mg , clarithromycin 500 mg and amoxicillin 1 gm BID before eating for 14 days ★
sucralfate [Carafate] (1g TAB; 1g/10ml susp) *Active duodenal ulcer:* 1g QID on a empty stomach; *Maintenance:* 1g Tab BID
sulfasalazine [Azulfidine] (Tab 500 mg) ADULTS 3-4g QD in evenly divided doses; PEDS 40-60 mg/kg/24h
Tritec [ranitidine bismuth citrate] (Tab 400 mg) Treatment of H. pylori: Tritec 400 mg BID on days 1-28, plus clarithromycin 500 mg TID on days 1-14
ursodiol [Actigall] (Cap 300 mg) 8-10 mg/kg/24h divided evenly into 2 or 3 daily doses
vasopressin [Pitressin Synthetic] (20 pressor units/ml inj) *Unlabeled use - To control GI bleeding:* 0.2-0.4 units/min IV/intra arterial (MAX 0.9 units/min)
orlistat [Xenical] (Cap 120 mg) 120 mg with or within 1 hour after each meal. *Lipase inhibitor* ★

GI Notes:

CONTRACEPTION

ORAL CONTRACEPTIVES (OC): Suppresses ovulation by altering the gonadotropin cycle. Also, alters the endometrial and endocervical cells creating a barrier to the sperm.

The following OC's are listed in order of increasing estrogen content

Monophasic	Progestin	Estrogen
Micronor	0.35mg norethindrone	NONE
Alesse	0.1mg levonorgestrel	
Levlite		ethinyl estradiol
Mircette	0.15mg desogestrel	20mcg
Loestrin 21 $^1/_{20}$, FE $^1/_{20}$	1mg norethindrone acetate	
Levlen, Levora, Nordette	0.15mg levonorgestrel	
Desogen, Ortho-cept	0.15mg desogestrel	ethinyl estradiol
LoOvral	0.3mg norgestrel	30mcg
Loestrin 21 $^{1.5}/_{30}$, FE $^{1.5}/_{30}$	1.5mg norethindrone acetate	
Demulen 1/35	1mg ethynodiol diacetate	
Ortho-Cyclen	0.25mg norgestimate	
Ovcon 35	0.4mg norethindrone	ethinyl estradiol
Nelova $^{0.5}/_{35}$E, Modicon, Genora $^{0.5}/_{35}$, Brevicon	0.5mg norethindrone	35mcg
Ortho-Novum $^1/_{35}$, Norinyl 1+35, Norethin $^1/_{35}$E, Nelova $^1/_{35}$E, N.E.E $^1/_{35}$, Genora $^1/_{35}$	1mg norethindrone	
Ovral	0.5mg norgestrel	
Demulen $^1/_{50}$	1mg ethynodiol diacetate	ethinyl estradiol
Ovcon 50		50mcg
Ortho-Novum $^1/_{50}$, Norinyl 1+50, Norethin $^1/_{50}$M, Nelova $^1/_{50}$M, Genora $^1/_{50}$	1mg norethindrone	Mestranol 50mcg

Biphasic	Days	Phase 1	Days	Phase 2
Ortho-Novum	10		11	
Nelova 10/11	10	0.5mg norethindrone/ 35mcg ethinyl estradiol	11	1mg norethindrone/ 35mcg ethinyl estradiol
Jenest-28	7		14	

Triphasic	Phase 1	Phase 2	Phase 3
Ortho TriCyclen	0.18mg norgestimate/ 35mcg ethinyl estradiol	0.215mg norgestimate/ 35mcg ethinyl estradiol	0.25mg norgestimate/ 35mcg ethinyl estradiol
Triphasil, Tri-Levlen	0.05mg levonorgestrel/ 30mcg ethinyl estradiol	0.075mg levonorgestrel/ 40mcg ethinyl estradiol	0.125mg levonorgestrel/ 30mcg ethinyl estradiol
Ortho-Novum 7/7/7	0.5mg norethindrone/ 35mcg ethinyl estradiol	0.75mg norethindrone/ 35mcg ethinyl estradiol	1mg norethindrone/ 35mcg ethinyl estradiol
Tri-Norinyl		1mg norethindrone/ 35mcg ethinyl estradiol	0.5mg norethindrone/ 35mcg ethinyl estradiol

Pharmacological effects of progestins				
	Androgen	Antiestrogen	Estrogen	Progestin
Norethynodrel	None	None	Pronounced	slight
Norethindrone	Moderate	Slight	Slight	slight
Norethindrone acetate	Moderate	Pronounced	Slight	slight
Ethynodiol Diacetate	Moderate	Slight	Slight	moderate
Norgestimate	None	Pronounced	None	pronounced
Desogestrel	none/slight	Pronounced	none/slight	pronounced
Norgestrel/levonorgestrel	Pronounced	Moderate	None	pronounced

Symptoms due to Oral Contraceptive Hormonal Levels			
Estrogen		Progestin	
Deficiency	Excess	Deficiency	Excess
Increased spotting Early or midcycle breakthrough bleeding Increased spotting	Edema, Nausea, Bloating, Migraine cephalgia, Hypertension, Cervical polyposis, Mucorrhea Melasma, Breast tenderness	Late breakthrough Bleeding Hypermenorrhea Amenorrhea	Weight gain, Fatigue Acne, oily scalp, Increased appetite, Hair loss, Hirsutism, Breast regression, Monilial vaginitis

Risks/Side effects: (in order of significance) Thromboembolism [relative risk (RI) compared to non-users 1.5-11], stroke [2-10], MI [2-6], hepatic neoplasm, possible associate with breast cancer, gall bladder disease. Risk is very low in women without underlying risk factors (HTN, obesity, diabetes, hyperlipidemia). Smoking cigarettes [5x risk for MI, 10-12x risk for stroke) and age > 35yoa increases risk. Potential for worsening asthma, HTN, carbohydrate intolerance, hyperlipidemia, epilepsy, worsening migraines, fibroids, nausea/vomiting, weight gain, depression, edema, amenorrhea and breakthrough bleeding.

Start new patients on ≤ 35mcg of estrogen.

Sunday start- start first Sunday after menstruation begins; *21 day regimen*- start on 5th day after menstrual bleeding begins; *28 day regimen*- includes 7 inert or iron containing tablets to take on last 7 days of cycle.

Contraindications: Absolute- history of thromboembolism/thrombophlebitis, atherosclerotic vascular disease, myocardial infarction, endometrial or breast cancer, impaired liver function or tumor, pregnancy, abnormal genital bleeding with unknown etiology, sickle cell anemia; Relative- Tobacco abuse, >35 years of age, hypertension, diabetes, hyperlipidemia, lactation, renal or heart disease.

Administration: Estrogen (ethinyl estradiol or mestranol 30-50mcg) and progestin (levonorgestrel or norethindrone compounds <1mg) combinations are used as fixed dosage or multiphasic for 21 days with a 7 day interval between packages. The pill should be started on the fifth day of the menstrual period. If two consecutive pills are missed, backup contraception should be used for the remainder of the course.

*Antibiotics may decrease the effectiveness of oral contraceptives, use backup method of contraception.

Other forms of Contraception:
- medroxyprogesterone [Depo-Provera 150 mg/ml] 150 mg IM every 3 months
- intrauterine device: SX: Increased menstrual flow, cramping and infection. Progesterone coating decreases symptoms. Requires replacement every 1-10 years. Relative contraindications: non-monogamous relationship, history of PID, heavy menstrual flow, dysmenorrhea.
- barrier/chemical: Condom, diaphragm, cervical cap, sponge and foam.
- sterilization: Tubal ligation should be considered permanent, although has 50% reversibility rate depending on type of procedure.
- Post-coital: Ovral 2 pills or LoOvral, Triphasil Ovral, Tri-Levlen, Nordette or Levlen 4 pills ASAP after unprotected intercourse (within 72h). Repeat dose 12h later. May treat with antiemetic with first dose then prn.

ENDOCRINOLOGY

AMENORRHEA: Primary- Pt has never menstruated. Failure to menstruate by age 18 or lack of breast development by 16y. DDX: Defect in reproductive tract, pituitary or gonadal failure or defects in sex steroidogenesis. DX: Physical exam, serum FSH and LH. TX: Steroid therapy or surgical correction. Secondary- No menses for 6 months with previous regular menses or 12 months of irregular menses. DDX: Pregnancy, menopause, weight loss, anorexia, anxiety, psychotropic drugs, polycystic ovarian disease, increased physical activity, hypothyroidism, pituitary adenoma or failure. DX: History, PE (signs of estrogen deficiency) radiological studies of sella turcica, progestin withdrawal test, thyroid studies, serum prolactin, FSH and LH. TX: Aimed at correcting normal cycle in the hypothalamic-pituitary-ovarian axis.

DYSMENORRHEA Due to increased prostaglandin release from endometrium. PRIMARY- No detectable organic basis. Onset usually at menarche. SX: Lower abdominal, spasmodic pain that may be associated with nausea, vomiting and diarrhea. Usually start at onset of menses, being most severe on the first and second day. SECONDARY- Due to pelvic lesion. DDX: Endometriosis, adenomyosis, PID, Ovarian cyst, IUD's. TX: NSAIDS (i.e. Indomethacin, Ibuprofen, mefenamic acid) for prostaglandin inhibition controls pain in 80% pts. Estrogen OC's (decreases prostaglandin synthesis by atrophy and decidualization of endometrium) may be used as primary therapy or combined with NSAIDS. Laparoscopy is indicated if no response after 4 months.

ENDOMETRIOSIS Menorrhagia, dyspareunia, or infertility caused by aberrant endometrial tissue. Usually 30-40yoa. 50% are asymptomatic. Two types: Internal endometriosis (Adenomyosis)- Diffuse extension of endometrial glands and stroma into myometrium; External endometriosis (endometriosis)- Glands and stromal implants outside the uterus. DX: History, physical exam, laparoscopy. TX: Hysterectomy or local excision. NSAIDS (i.e. Indomethacin, Ibuprofen, mefenamic acid) or Danazol may be beneficial.

HIRSUTISM: Most commonly familial. If rapid onset think ovarian or adrenal tumor. DX: Prolactin, testosterone and dehydroepiandrosterone serum radioimmunoassays.

MENOPAUSE: Lack of menses for one year in pt with previous regular cycles. Premature if <35yr. Symptoms due to estrogen deprivation. SX: Hot flushes, mood changes, night sweats, vaginal dryness, urinary urgency, headaches, dyspareunia. TX: Estrogen replacement for 25 days with progestin supplementation (to protect endometrium from neoplastic changes) 10-12 days at the end of the cycle. Non-cyclic replacement (estrogen only)- get U/S or endometrial bx if bleeding after 1-6 months. Combined estrogen and progesterone now available- see *Hormones in the Endocrinology section*.

PREMENSTRUAL SYNDROME (PMS): Thought to be due to increased prolactin late in the menstrual cycle. Bromocriptine and progesterone may be helpful.

PUBERTY: Onset 12 yoa, duration 4-5 years. Menarche 13yoa average. Sequence of events: accelerated growth →breast budding→ pubic hair→ axillary hair.

INFECTIOUS DISEASE

BACTERIAL VAGINOSIS: Malodorous vaginal discharge, pH 5-6. Associated with Gardnerella vaginalis. DX: "clue" cells on wet prep, "Fishy" odor with KOH. TX: metronidazole 0.5 gm BID x7 days or 0.75% vaginal gel BID x 5 days. Not thought to be sexually transmitted.

CHLAMYDIA TRACHOMATIS: Most common STD in the US. Most common in unmarried, promiscuous, young, indigent women. Dyspareunia, discharge, spotting DX: Chlamydiazyme, Mucopurulent cervicitis (yellowish endocervical secretion with PMNs), cervical friability. TX: doxycycline 100mg BID for 7 days, or azithromycin (Zithromax) 1gm single dose. Also treat partner.

GONORRHEA: SX: Dysuria, suprapubic pain, menorrhagia, spotting, purulent discharge. DX: Thayer-Martin culture or Gonozyme. TX: Ceftriaxone 250mg IM single dose + doxycycline 100mg BID or tetracycline 500mg PO QID for 7 days or azithromycin 2gm single dose. Also treat partner. Repeat cultures 1-2 months.

HERPES: First episode usually painful vesicular or ulcerative genital lesions, dysuria, fever, malaise. DX: exam, viral cultures, Tzanck test. TX: Acyclovir 400 mg PO TID or 200mg 5x/dfor 10 days decreases symptoms and shortens viral shedding in primary attacks of HSV I & II. Vaginal childbirth after TX only if negative weekly cultures. May treat recurrent episodes with 5 day course

HIV: see *Infectious Disease section*. Often presents in females with invasive carcinoma or recurrent monilial vaginitis

HUMAN PAPILLOMAVIRUS: Accounts for the majority of abnormal PAP smears. Types 16, 18, 31, 33, 35 are associated with invasive cancers and 6 & 8 with Condyloma acuminatum. DX: PAP smear, colposcopy. TX: Podophyllin apply for 4h q wk until gone or Trichloroacetic acid 30-50% 2-3/wk then wash with soap & water.

MONILIAL VAGINITIS: "Cheesy white" discharge, pH 4.5, pruritus. TX: see vaginal antifungals below. Frequently follow antibiotic treatment. Check glucose and HIV status if recurrent.

PELVIC INFLAMMATORY DISEASE (PID): Cervical, adnexal and abdominal tenderness, fever. DX: Chlamydiazyme, GC & chlamydia culture, CBC. TX: Ceftriaxone 250 mg IM/IV single dose + doxycycline 100 mg PO BID for 14 days or ofloxaxin 300 mg PO BID + flagyl 500 mg BID (or clindamycin 300mg QID) for 14 days

SYPHILIS: Transmission requires exposure to cutaneous or mucosal lesions. Incubation is 10-90 days. Chancre (Condylomata latum) is a papule that erodes and ulcerates and is usually painless and on the genitalia. DX: RPR, VDRL & FTA-absorption. TX: Benzathine Penicillin G 2.4 million units IM or Tetracycline 500 mg PO QID x 15d.

SEPTIC PELVIC THROMBOPHLEBITIS: Diagnosis of exclusion. Recurrent spiking temperature despite antimicrobial coverage. TX: IV heparin and antibiotic for 7 days.

TRICHOMONAL VAGINITIS: Foul smelling, "frothy", clear-greenish discharge, trichomonads on wet prep, pH 5-7. TX: Pt and partner with metronidazole.

VAGINAL ANTI-INFECTIVES

clotrimazole OTC [Gyne-Lotrimin] (Cream 1%, Tab 100, 500 mg) cream topical apply BID or vaginal 1 applicatorful q HS for 7d, Vaginal tab 100 mg q HS for 7d or 500 mg at HS for 1 d
fluconazole [Diflucan] (Tab 50,100,150,200mg) PO 150mg single dose for vaginal candidiasis
miconazole OTC [Monistat] (Cream 2%, Supp 100, 200 mg) cream 1 applicatorful q HS for 7d, vaginal Supp 100 mg for 7d or 200 mg for 3d
metronidazole [MetroGel-Vaginal] (Gel 0.75%) 1 applicatorful BID for 5 days
nystatin (Tab 100000u) 1 vaginal tab daily for 2 weeks
terconazole [Terazol] (Cream 0.4, 0.8%, Supp 80mg) Cream q HS 0.4% for 7d, 0.8% for 3d; Supp q HS for 3d
tioconazole [Vagistat-1] (Oint 6.5%) 1 applicatorful at HS
triple sulfa [Sultrin] (cream, supp) 1 applicatorful BID for 4-6d, 1 tab BID for 10d

GYNECOLOGY 59

INFERTILITY
COUPLE FACTOR: Evaluate intercourse techniques, timing and frequency. **MALE FACTOR:** Problem identified 40% of the time. Evaluated by semen analysis. **FEMALE FACTOR:** Ovulation established by Basal Body Temperature. Postcoital test to evaluate cervical mucous quality and quantity. Laparoscopy to identify endometriosis. Hysterosalpingogram to identify intrauterine abnormalities.

ONCOLOGY
BREAST CARCINOMA: Most common female cancer. Second to lung cancer in mortality. *Risks-* family history, menarche <12 yoa, nulliparity, obesity, endometrial cancer, first pregnancy >35yoa. Metastases to bone, lung or liver. Usually diagnosed after painless lump is found. *Signs-* nipple retraction, elevation, inversion or bloody discharge, skin dimpling, "orange peeling", supraclavicular & axillary lymphadenopathy. DX: mammogram (Pts with family history should be screened annually after 35yoa or >50yoa if no family history.

CERVICAL CARCINOMA: Average age at diagnosis 45yr. Dysplasia and CIS, which are precursors to invasive carcinoma, can be detected by PAP smear. Annual PAP smears are recommended when sexually active and from age 18. 60% die from complications of local spread (i.e. Uremia due to ureter obstruction from tumor), 35% die from sepsis. 1/3 have metastasis to lung, spleen and liver. 87% are squamous cell and 13% are adenocarcinoma. SX: Postmenopausal, postcoital & intermenstrual bleeding and discharge are the most common for invasive cancer. Risk factors: high parity, STD's, multiple & uncircumcised sex partners, family history, early intercourse, HPV type 16 or 18, cervical dysplasia or CIS.

PAP SMEAR CYTOPATHOLOGY REPORTING SYSTEMS

Class System	WHO System	CIN System	Bethesda System
I	Normal	Normal	Within Normal Limits
II	Inflammation		Other (Infection, Reactive & reparative)
III	Dysplasia		Squamous intraepithelial lesions
	Mild	CIN-1	
	Moderate	CIN-2	Low grade
	Severe		High grade
IV	Carcinoma in situ	CIN-3	
V	Invasive squamous cell Ca	Invasive squamous cell Ca	Squamous cell Ca
	Adenocarcinoma	Adenocarcinoma	Adenocarcinoma

ENDOMETRIAL CARCINOMA: Most common pelvic carcinoma. Risk factors: advancing age, diabetes, obesity, low parity. SX: post menopausal bleeding. DX: Endometrial biopsy or D&C. Staging: Ia- confined to corpus, sounds <8cm; Ib- confined to corpus, sounds >8cm; II- involves cervix and corpus; IIIA- extends outside uterus but confined to true pelvis.

OVARIAN CARCINOMA: Most common cause of death by gynecologic malignancy. SX: Abdominal mass, pain, ascites. Decreased risk with OC use and high parity.

VULVAR CARCINOMA: Peak incidence in the 7th decade. Local and lymphatic spread. Squamous cell 70% Epidermoid 25%, Melanoma 4%. SX: Pruritus, ulcer, lump or bleeding.

GYNECOLOGIC MALIGNANCIES, STAGING & SURVIVAL

Stage	Ovarian	% 5-Yr Survival	Endometrial	% 5-Yr Survival	Cervix	% 5-Yr Survival
0					Carcinoma in situ	100
I	Confined to ovary	90	Confined to corpus	89	Confined to uterus	85
II	Confined to pelvis	70	Involves corpus & cervix	80	Invades beyond uterus but not to pelvic wall	60
III	Intraabdominal Spread	15-20	Extends outside uterus but not outside true pelvis	30	Extends to pelvic wall and/or Lower 1/3 or vagina, or hydronephrosis	33
IV	Spread outside Abdomen	1-5	Extends outside true pelvis or involves bladder or rectum	9	Invades mucosa of bladder or rectum or extends beyond true pelvis	7

MISCELLANEOUS

<u>capecitabine</u> [Xeloda] oral anti-neoplastic for metastatic breast cancer

<u>Plan B</u> [progestogen emergency contraceptives] (Tab 0.75 mg levonorgestrel) 1 tab PO within 72 hrs after unprotected intercourse, then the second tab 12 hrs after the first dose ★

<u>Prometrium</u> [progesterone](Cap 100 mg) see package insert for dosing

<u>tamoxifen</u> [Nolvadex] (Tab 10 mg) PO 10-20 mg BID

<u>Taxol/Platinol</u> AQ [Paclitaxel/cisplatin] approved for 1st line and subsequent therapy for advanced ovarian carcinoma

<u>toremifene</u> (Fareston) (Tab 60 mg) antiestrogen for breast cancer, 60 mg QD until disease progression is observed

<u>trastuzumab</u> [Herceptin] (Powder 440 mg) 4 mg/kg infused over 90 minutes; Weekly maintenance dose is 2 mg/kg and can be infused over 30 minutes. *Breast cancer* ★

<u>Zoladex</u> [goserelin acetate/futamide] (3.6 mg) indication for endometrial thinning

GYN Notes:

MORPHOLOGIC CLASSIFICATION OF ANEMIA
MACROCYTIC (MCV>100)
- **Megaloblastic:** *vitamin B_{12} deficiency (pernicious anemia), folic acid deficiency (nutritional, sprue, etc.), inherited disorders of DNA synthesis (orotic aciduria), drug-induced disorders of DNA synthesis (chemotherapeutic agents, anticonvulsants, oral contraceptives).*
- **Nonmegaloblastic:** *accelerated erythropoiesis (Hemolytic anemia), increased membrane surface area-response to hemorrhage*

MICROCYTIC (MCV<80)
Iron deficiency (Chronic blood loss, poor diet, decreased absorption), disorders of globin synthesis, disorders of porphyrin & heme synthesis (Pyridoxine-responsive).

Comparison of Microcytic/Hypochromic Anemias

	Iron def anemia	βThalassemia trait	Anemia of chronic disease	Sideroblastic anemia
Serum Iron	↓	N	↓	↑
TIBC	↑	N	↓	N
Serum ferritin	↓	N	↑	↑
RBC protoporphyrin	↑	N	↑	↑
Hgb A_2	↓	↑	N	↓

Stages of Iron Deficiency

	Normal	Mild	Moderate	Severe
Hemoglobin g%	15.0	13.0	10.0	5.0
MCV	N	↓	↓	↓↓
MCHC	N	N	↓	↓↓
Marrow Fe stores	↑	↓	↓	↓
Serum Fe/TIBC μg/L	1000/3000	750/3000	500/4500	250/6000

NORMOCYTIC (MCV 81-99)
Recent blood loss, hypervolemia (pregnancy), hemolytic dz., hypoplastic bone marrow (aplastic anemia), infiltrated bone marrow (myelofibrosis, leukemia), endocrine abnormality (hypothyroid, hypoadrenal), chronic disorders, renal dz., liver dz.

BLOOD & BLOOD PRODUCTS
POTENTIAL COMPLICATIONS
<u>Hemolytic transfusion rxn:</u> *Immediate* - shock, chills, fever, dyspnea, chest &/or back pain, HA, &/or abnormal bleeding, DIC (may result in death). Hemoglobinemia, hemoglobinuria, ↑ bilirubin. Stop transfusion, treat shock & renal failure with fluids & diuretics. *Delayed* - signs may be sudden ↓ Hgb or persistent anemia despite transfusions, fever, hemoglobinuria, &/or ↑bilirubin. May have +direct Coombs. Usually benign course.

<u>Infectious disease:</u> Hepatitis B & C, HIV-1, HIV-2, HTLV-1, CMV are routinely screened for (ALT screening is no longer routine). Screening tests eliminate most, but not all, posttransfusion hepatitis. Rare - brucella, toxoplasma, Colorado tick fever, Bartonella, Babesia, Borrelia, parvovirus, plasmodia, Leishmania, Epstein-Barr, and certain trypanosomes.

<u>Bacterial contamination</u> of components is rare. May be gram negative bacteria with endotoxins. Consider when pt develops chills, high fever, or hypotension during or immediately after transfusion.

<u>Alloimmunization:</u> May occur to RBC, WBC, platelets, or protein antigens. Usually not immediate rxn; creates positive antibody screen on subsequent testing.

<u>Graft vs. Host:</u> May occur in children & adults with underdeveloped or impaired immune systems due to lymphocytes in cellular blood products. Irradiated products reduce the risk.

<u>Febrile rxns:</u> ≈1% of transfusions. Usually caused by antibodies that agglutinate leukocytes.

<u>Allergic rxns:</u> Urticaria, wheezing, or angioedematous rxns in ≈1%. Premedicate with antihistamines may help. *Anaphylactoid rxns* - bronchospasm, dyspnea, pulmonary edema with IgA antibodies. Treat with epi & steroids. Use frozen or washed cells, & IgA-deficient plasma.

<u>Circulatory overload</u> may result in pulmonary edema. PRBC's typically contain ≈8-20mEq Na^+/unit (if Adenine-saline is added, PRBC's contain ≈24-30mEq Na^+/unit).

<u>Iron overload</u> may result in hemosiderosis. Occurs in pt's given repeated transfusions over long periods.

<u>Significant depletion of coag proteins</u> & platelets is rare. Consider DIC if excessive bleeding occurs.

<u>Microaggregates</u> ≈170-260 μm will usually be trapped in the microaggregate filter.

<u>Metabolic complications</u> with large amounts (≥pt's blood volume) of transfusion which are rapidly infused, or if severe liver or kidney disease is present. *Hypothermia*: risk of cardiac arrhythmias with rapid infusion of cold blood. Blood warmers are preventative. *Citrate toxicity*: Rare. Complexing of Ca^{2+} by anticoagulant. *Acidosis*: occurs with massive transfusions, rarely requires treatment. Citrate is rapidly converted to HCO_3 & pyruvate. *Alterations in K^+*: ↑ K possible with continued or massive transfusions. ↓K with citrate-induced met acidosis.

WHOLE BLOOD

Use for symptomatic anemia with large volume deficit. Must be ABO-identical. Labile coag factors deteriorate in 24h after collection. Infuse as fast as the pt can tolerate.

PACKED RED BLOOD CELLS (PRBCs)

Contain ≈ 300 ml/unit with Hct of 65-80%. ↑ O$_2$-carrying capacity of blood. Indicated for virtually all pt's with symptomatic ↓ O$_2$- carrying capacity, exchange transfusions (use PRBC's <7days old), & to restore blood volume after hemorrhage. Contraindicated when anemia can be corrected with specific medications or in coag deficiency. PRBC's can be used when ABO-compatible, but not ABO-identical. Give as fast as pt tolerates. Adenine-Saline (AS) may be added to lower the Hct to 55-65%. Use if volume deficit present. AS-1 & AS-5 contain mannitol, AS-3 contains citrate & phosphate without mannitol. The label indicates which AS was used. May have leukocytes removed for use in febrile reactions from leukocyte antibodies.

FRESH FROZEN PLASMA (FFP)

Plasma which has been frozen within 8h after collection of whole blood. Contains ≈200 units of Factor VIII plus all other labile & stable coagulation factors. Should be ABO-compatible. Infuse in <4h. Use within 24h after thawing (stored @ 1-6°C). Use is limited to bleeding pt's who require replacement of labile coag factors when simultaneous blood volume expansion is required & in Thrombotic Thrombocytopenic Purpura (TTP).

CRYOPRECIPITATE AHF

Contains ≥80 units of Factor VIII (FVIII:C) & ≥150mg fibrinogen in <15ml plasma. Also, contains Factor XIII, von Willebrand Factor (AHF-vWF), & fibronectin. Use to control bleeding associated with Factor VIII deficiency, von Willebrand's disease, or to replace fibrinogen or Factor XIII. Use only when lab tests indicate a specific coag defect for which this product is indicated. Compatibility testing is unnecessary. ABO-compatible units are preferred (Rh compatible not necessary).For treatment of bleeding in hemophilia A. Response may be less then expected, depending on extravascular space saturation. Monitor response with Factor VIII:C assays. Von Willebrand's disease requires smaller amounts. Monitor fibrinogen levels in treatment of hypofibrinogenemia.

$$\text{Number of bags of cryoprecipitate required} = \frac{\text{[desired FVIII:C level(\%) x patient's plasma volume (ml)]}}{\text{avg. units of FVIII:C per bag of cryoprecipitate}}$$

PLATELETS, CONCENTRATE

Contains ≈5.5X10^{10} platelets suspended in 40-70ml of plasma. May contain trace amounts of RBC's in some bags (Rh+ units may possibly sensitize Rh- child-bearing age females). Use ABO-compatible platelets (ABO-incompatible platelets may cause a + direct Coombs & a low grade hemolysis. One bag of platelets is expected to raise the platelet count of a 70kg adult by 5-10 X 10^9/L & increase the count of an 18kg child by 20 X 10^9/L or more. Response will be less in the presence of sepsis, fever or ITP, previously alloimmunized by previous transfusions, when platelets are consumed (e.g., DIC), or when they are being sequestered (e.g., splenomegaly). Monitor the response with a platelet count 1-2h after transfusion. The usual dose in an adult is 6-8 bags. Transfuse as fast as tolerated.

PLATELETS, PHERESIS

Hemapheresis harvests a therapeutic adult dose of platelets from a single donor (contains >3 X 10^{11} platelets/bag in a total volume of 200-500 ml). One pheresis bag is ≈ 5-8 bags of platelet concentrate. Use is the same as described for platelet concentrate.

GRANULOCYTES, PHERESIS

Hemapheresis units of granulocytes also contain large numbers of other leukocytes, platelets, & RBC's. Usual volume is 200-300 ml of anticoagulant & plasma. The infusion of granulocytes rarely changes the pt's WBC count. Serologic compatibility testing must be performed due to the high number of RBC's.

BLOOD MODIFIERS/MISC

aminocaproic acid [Amicar] (250 mg/ml inj; 250, 500 mg TAB; 250 mg/cc syrup) Initially, 5g PO/IV, followed by 1-1.25 g q1h (MAX 30g/24h). *Inhibits plasminogen activator substances & plasmin.*

antihemophilic factor (Factor VIII; AHF) [Helixate, Kogenate, Recombinate] (actual # of AHF units are indicated on the vial) *AHF/IU required = body wt(kg) X desired factor VIII ↑ (% normal) X 0.5*

anti-inhibitor coagulant complex [Autoplex T, Feiba VH] 25-100 Factor VIII correctional units/kg IV q6-12h. *Contains variable amts. of activated & precursor clotting factors, & kinin generating system factors. Use in Factor VIII deficient pts who have laboratory-measurable inhibitors to Factor VIII.*

antithrombin III (human) [Thrombate III] (5000 IU): dose per the following equation:

$$\text{Dosage units} = \frac{\text{[desired ATIII level(\%) - baseline ATIII level(\%)] x patient's body weight (kg)]}}{1\%/(\text{IU/bag})}$$

<u>Coagulation Factor VIIa</u> (Recombinant) [NovoSeven] (1.2, 4.8 mg/vial) 90 mcg/kg given IVP every 2 hours until hemostasis is achieved, typically 35 and 120 mcg/kg. *hemophilia A or B patients with inhibitors to Factor VIII or IX* ★

<u>epoetin alfa</u> (erythropoietin; EPO) [Epogen, Procrit] (Vials 2000, 3000, 4000, 10000 units/cc) *Anemia* - dosage varies depending on underlying cause of anemia.

<u>desmopressin</u> [DDAVP, Stimate] (Inj 4 mcg/ml; NS 10 mcg/spray; Nasal Sol 0.1, 1.5 mg/ml) *Hemophilia A & Von Willebrand's* 0.3 mcg/kg IV in saline (50 ml if >10 kg, 10 ml if <10kg) over 15-30min; OR *>50 kg use* 150 mcg intranasally each nostril single dose, *<50kg use* 75 mcg intranasally each nostril single dose

<u>hydroxyurea</u> [Droxia] (Cap 200 mg) initial dose 15 mg/kg/day as a single dose. Blood count must be monitored every two weeks (approved for the reduction of the frequency of painful crises and the need for transfusions in adult sickle-cell anemia patients with recurrent moderate-to-severe painful crises)

<u>Factor IX complex (human)</u> [Konyne 80, Profilnine SD, Proplex T] Formula is guide only: Units required = 1 unit/kg X body wt(kg) X desired increase(% of normal; min 20%) *Contains* Factors IX, II, VII, X. *Factor VII deficiency* Proplex T <u>only</u>.

<u>filgrastim</u> (Granulocyte Colony Stimulating Factor; G-CSF) [Neupogen] (300 µg/ml) *Myelosuppressive chemo-* SC/IV 5 mcg/kg/day given >24h before or after administration of chemotherapy, for up to 2 wks until ANC >10,000mm^3. *Bone marrow transplant-* SC 24h infusion or IV 4-24h infusion 10mcg/kg/day at least 24h after chemotherapy or bone marrow infusion

<u>imiglucerase</u> (Cerezyme) *Gaucherie's disease* (anemia, thrombocytopenia, bone disease, hepatosplenomegaly) IV initial 2.5 U/kg 3 times a week, up to 60 U/kg q 1-4wks, Maintenance: progressive reductions at 3-6 month intervals

<u>sargramostim</u> (Granulocyte Macrophage Colony Stimulating Factor; GM-CSF) [Leukine, Prokine] (250, 500 µg) *Myeloid reconstitution after autologous bone marrow transplant, OR bone marrow transplant failure or engraftment delay* use 250 µg/m^2/day as a 2h IV infusion.

<u>tranexamic acid</u> [Cyklokapron] (500 mg TAB; 100 mg/ml inj) 10 mg/kg IV prior to tooth extraction, then 25 mg/kg PO TID/QID X 2-8 days after surgery; *Alternative:* 25 mg/kg PO TID/QID beginning 1 day prior to surgery. *Competitive inhibitor of plasminogen activation, & noncompetitive inhibition of plasmin.*

Hematology Notes:

CHEMOPROPHYLAXIS AFTER OCCUPATIONAL EXPOSURE TO HIV
(Adapted from MMWR, vol 45, num 22, pg 471)

Exposure type	Source material	Prophylaxis	Regimen[b]
Percutaneous	Blood[c]		
	Highest risk	Recommend[a]	ZDV + 3TC + IDV
	Increased risk	Recommend	ZDV + 3TC +/- IDV[e]
	No increased risk	Offer	ZDV + 3TC
	Fluid containing visible blood, other		
	potentially infectious fluid, or tissue	Offer	ZDV + 3TC
	Other body fluid (e.g., urine)	Not offer	none
Mucous membrane	Blood	Offer	ZDV + 3TC +/- IDV
	Fluid containing visible blood, other		
	potentially infectious fluid[d], or tissue	Offer	ZDV + 3TC
	Other body fluid (e.g., urine)	Not offer	None
Skin, increased risk[f]	Blood	Offer	ZDV + 3TC +/- IDV
	Fluid containing visible blood, other		
	potentially infectious fluid, or tissue	Offer	ZDV + 3TC
	Other body fluid (e.g., urine)	Not offer	none

[a]*Recommend* – Postexposure prophylaxis (PEP) recommended with counseling. *Offer* – PEP offered with counseling. *Not offer* – These are not occupational exposures.

[b]*Regimens*: zidovudine (ZVD) 200 mg TID; lamivudine (3TC) 150 mg BID; indinavir (IDV) 800 mg TID (may use saquinavir 600 mg TID if IDV not available). Prophylaxis for 4 weeks.

[c]*Highest risk* – BOTH larger vol. Of blood (e.g. deep injury with large diameter hollow needle previously in pt's vein or artery) AND blood containing high titer of HIV (e.g. source with acute retroviral illness or end-stage AIDS; viral load measurements may be considered, but have not been evaluated). *Increased risk* – EITHER exposure to a larger volume of blood OR blood with a higher titer of HIV.

[d]Includes semen, vaginal secretions, CSF, synovial, pleural, pericardial, peritoneal & amniotic fluid.

[e]Possible toxicity of additional drug may not be warranted.

[f]Skin ↑risk is for high titer of HIV, prolonged contact, an extensive area, or where skin integrity is visibly compromised. Without ↑risk, the risk of drug toxicity outweighs benefit of PEP.

HIV INFECTION CRITERIA: Persons ≥ 13 yrs with repeatedly (≥ 2) reactive screening tests (ELISA) + specific antibodies identified by a supplemental test (Western blot - CDC criteria for reactive pattern =). Other specific methods of diagnosis include virus isolation, antigen detection, and PCR detection of HIV genetic material.

REQUIRED DISEASE PROPHYLAXIS FOR HIV PATIENTS
All HIV pts: Tuberculosis (ppd >5mm; prior untreated +ppd; contact with case of active TB; probable exposure to INH or multi-drug resistant TB.) *Symptomatic* or *Asymptomatic with CD4 ≤500/mm³ or >30-50,000 HIV RNA copies/ml*: Begin antiretroviral Tx. *Asymptomatic with >5-10,000 HIV RNA copies/ml*: Consider antiretroviral Tx. *CD4 ≤200mm³*: PCP & Herpes Simplex 1&2. *CD4 ≤100mm³*: Toxoplasma gondii with + antibody titer. *CD4 ≤75mm³*: Mycobacterium Avium-Intracellulare. *CD4 ≤ 50mm³*: CMV & cryptococcus.

NUCLEOSIDE ANALOGUES
Combivir (Tab lamivudine 150 mg + zidovudine 300mg) *>12 yoa & ≥ 50 kg* use 1 tab PO BID
Didanosine [Videx] (Chew Tabs 25/50/100/150 mg, powder for solution Adults 100/167/250/375 mg/packet, Pediatric 2/4g/bottle): see package. *Major side effects*: pancreatitis & peripheral neuropathy
lamivudine [Epivir] (Tab 150 mg) 1 tab PO BID in combination with Retrovir. *Major side effects*: well tolerated. [Epivir-HBV] (Tab 100 mg, Sol 5 mg/ml) *treatment of chronic hepatitis B* – 100 mg PO QD ★
stavudine [d4T, Zerit] (Caps 15, 20, 30, 40 mg) advanced HIV who are intolerant to other therapies. Initial ≥60kg 40 mg q12h, <60kg 30 mg q12h. Side effect: peripheral neuropathy
Zalcitabine [HIVID, formerly ddC] (Tab 0.375, 0.750 mg) 0.750 mg + 200 mg zidovudine q8h. *Major side effects*: Sensorimotor peripheral neuropathy
Zidovudine [RETROVIR, formerly AZT] (Tab 100 mg, Syr 50 mg/5ml) 600 mg/D, 200 mg q8h or 100 mg q4h. [RETROVIR IV] (10 mg/cc): 1-2 mg/kg over 1h q4h. *Major side effects*: granulocytopenia & anemia

NON-NUCLEOSIDE REVERSE TRANSCRIPTASE INHIBITORS
delavirdine [Rescriptor] (Tab 100 mg) *Adults ≥16yoa* 400 mg PO TID. Must use with nucleoside analogue or protease inhibitor. *Major side effects*: rash
efavirenz [Sustiva] (Cap 50, 100, 200 mg) *Adults & children >3yoa & >40lbs* use 600 mg QD with a PI or NRTI with or without food; for children <40lbs see package insert. Category C ★

<u>nevirapine</u> [Viramune] (Tab 200 mg; Susp 50 mg/5 ml) *Peds (2 mos-8 yrs)* 4 mg/kg QD for 14 dys followed by 7 mg/kg twice daily. *>8 yoa* - 4 mg/kg QD for 14 days followed by 4 mg/kg twice daily. ★ Adjunctive agent, 200 mg for 14 days followed by 200 mg twice daily with a nucleoside analogue antiretroviral agent

PROTEASE INHIBITORS

<u>abacavir Sulfate</u> [Ziagen] (Tab 300 mg; Sol 20 mg/ml) 300 mg BID in combination with other antiretroviral agents. *Peds (3 mos - 16 yoa):* 8 mg/kg BID (Max 300 mg BID) ★
<u>amprenavir</u> HIV [Agenerase] (Cap 50, 150 mg; Sol 15 mg/ml) ★
<u>indinavir</u> [Crixivan] (Cap 200, 400 mg) 800 mg PO 1h before or 2h after meals q8h. *Major side effects:* nephrolithiasis & asymptomatic hyperbilirubinemia
<u>nelfinavir</u> [Viracept] (Tab 250 mg) *Adults >13yoa* 750 mg PO TID. *Peds 2-13yoa* 20-30 mg/kg PO TID, Max 750 mg/D. *Major side effects:* diarrhea, nausea, flatus, abdominal pain, and rash
<u>ritonavir</u> [Norvir] (Tab 100 mg, Oral Sol 600 mg/7.5ml)PO with meals 600 mg BID
<u>saquinavir</u> [Fortovase] (Caps 200 mg) *>16yoa* use 1.2 g (6 caps) PO TID within 2 hrs after meal
<u>saquinavir</u> [Invirase] (Cap 200 mg) *≥16yoa* 600 mg within 2h after a full meal. *Major side effects:* diarrhea, abdominal discomfort, and nausea

AIDS RELATED COMPLEX (ARC) THERAPEUTIC AGENTS

<u>acyclovir sodium</u> [Zovirax for IV only] (500 mg per 10ml vials, 1000 mg per 20ml vials) *Mucosal & Cutaneous HSV in immunocompromised Pts* - 5 mg/kg IV over 1h q8h X 7D; *Severe initial clinical Genital Herpes* - same as previous for 5 days; *Herpes Simplex Encephalitis & Varicella Zoster in immunocompromised Pts* - 10 mg/kg over 1h q8h X 7d; Wts are Ideal Body Weight. For children under 12 yoa: *Mucosal & Cutaneous HSV in immunocompromised Pts* - 250 mg/m² IV over 1h q8h X 7d; *Herpes Simplex Encephalitis & Varicella Zoster in immunocompromised Pts* - 500 m/m² over 1h q8h X 7d.
<u>alitretinoin</u> [Panretin] (Gel 0.1%) Initially apply BID, may increase gradually to 3-4 times daily. (60g) *Kaposi's sarcoma cutaneous lesions* Preg D ★
<u>atovaquone</u> [Mepron] (Tab 250 mg) *Pneumocystis carinii pneumonia* - 750 mg PO TID with food x 21 days.
<u>azithromycin</u> [Zithromax] for prevention of MAC in advanced HIV infection, PO 250-500 mg qd, 1200 mg/week
<u>cidofovir</u> [Vistide] treatment of CMV retinitis in AIDS patients 5 mg/kg IV over 1 h once a week for 2 weeks. Must be given with probenecid and IV saline.
<u>dronabinol</u> [Marinol] (2.5, 5, 10 mg Tabs) *appetite stimulant:* initially 2.5 mg BID ac (MAX 20 mg/day); *anti-emetic:* 5 mg/m² 1-3h before chemo, then _ 2-4h (4-6 times/day).
<u>epoetin alfa</u> [Epogen, Procrit] (Vials 2000, 3000, 4000, 10000 units/cc) *Anemia* - dosage varies.
<u>famciclovir</u> [Famvir] (Tab 125, 250, 500 mg) *Herpes Zoster* - 500 mg q8h X 7D; *Genital Herpes* - 125 mg q12h X 5d. Adjust for CrCl.
<u>fluconazole</u> [Diflucan] (Tab 50, 100, 200 mg; Inj 200 mg/100cc & 400 mg/200cc) *Candidiasis* - 200-400 mg PO/IV day 1, then 100-200 mg/day x 2 weeks. *Cryptococcal meningitis* - 400 mg PO/IV day 1, then 200 mg/day x 10-12 weeks. PO dose is equal to IV.
<u>fluoxymesterone</u> [Halotestin] (Tab 2, 5, 10 mg) *Weight loss* 10 mg PO BID.
<u>fomivirsen</u> [Vitravene] (Inj 6.6 mg/ml, Single dose vial 0.25 ml) Initial 0.05 ml intravitreal injection into the affected eye following application of standard topical or local anesthetics and antimicrobials using a 30-gauge needle on a low-volume (eg, tuberculin) syringe every other week for 2 doses then maintenance doses once every 4 weeks
<u>foscarnet sodium</u> [Foscavir] (24 mg/cc in 500 & 250 ml glass bottles) *CMV retinitis* - dosage varies.
<u>ganciclovir sodium</u> [Cytovene] (Cap 250 mg; Vial 500 mg) *CMV retinitis* -Induction IV 5 mg/kg over 1h q12h for 14-21 days then maintenance once daily. PO maintenance 1000 mg TID with food
<u>interferon alfa-2b recombinant</u> [Intron A, Roferon-A] (Vials 3, 9, 18, 36 million IU) *AIDS related Kaposi's sarcoma*
<u>intravenous immune serum globulin</u> [IVIG, Gamimune] (2.5gms) *Parvovirus B19* 400 mg/kg/D X 10D.
<u>megestrol acetate</u> [Megace] (Susp 40 mg/ml) *Anorexia* 800 mg PO qd.
<u>nandrolone</u> [Durabolin] (25, 50, 100, 200 mg/ml) *Anorexia:* 100 mg IM q week.
<u>pentamidine isethionate</u> [NebuPent, Pentam 300] (Vials 300 mg per single dose) *Pneumocystis carinii pneumonia* -300 mg nebulized q week for prophylaxis; 300 mg IM/IV QD x 14 days for treatment.
<u>rifabutin</u> [Mycobutin] (Cap 150 mg) *Mycobacterium avium complex prophylaxis* - 300 mg PO QD.
<u>RHO immune globulin</u> [RhoGAM] *Thrombocytopenia*- 25-50mcg/kg/D X 1 Wk; repeat infusions q3 Wks
<u>Testosterone</u> [Everone] (100, 200 mg/ml) 200-400 mg IM q2 weeks.
<u>TMP/SMX</u> [Bactrim] (Tab 80 mg TMP + 200 mg SMX; DS 160 mg TMP + 800 mg SMX; Susp 40 mg TMP + 200 mg SMX/5cc) *Pneumocystis carinii pneumonia* - 20 mg/kg TMP & 100 mg/kg SMX per 24h divided into PO/IVPB q6h doses X 14 days.
<u>valacyclovir</u> [Valtrex] (Cap 500 mg) *Herpes Zoster* - 2 caps (1g) TID X 7 days; *Recurrent Genital Herpes* - 1 cap BID X 5 days.

AMINOGLYCOSIDES & COMBINATIONS

(*Ototoxicity* - Streptomycin=Kanamycin>Amikacin=gentamicin=tobramycin>netilmicin; *Renal toxicity* - kanamycin=amikacin=gentamicin=netilmicin>tobramycin>streptomycin)

Peak(P): 30(IV)-60(IM)mins after infusion; Trough(T): just prior to next dose.

<u>amikacin</u> [Amikin] (Vials 250 mg/cc, 100 mg/2cc, 500 mg/2cc, 1 g/4cc) 15 mg/kg/24h IM/IV in 2-3 divided doses. For IV, infuse over 30-60 mins. *P:* <35 μg/ml, *T:* <10 μg/ml.

<u>gentamicin</u> [Garamycin] (Vials 80 mg/2cc, 60 mg/1.5cc, 20 mg/2cc) *ADULTS use* 1 mg/kg q8h (3 mg/kg/24h) *P:* 4-6 μg/ml; *T:* <2 μg/ml; *CHILDREN* 2-2.5 mg/kg q8h; *INFANTS & NEONATES* 2.5 mg/kg q8h; *PREMATURE or FULL-TERM NEONATES* ≤1 WEEK OF AGE 2.5 mg/kg q12h; *P:* 3-5 μg/ml; *T:* <2 μg/ml.

<u>kanamycin</u> [Kantrex] (75 mg, 500 mg, 1g inj) 15 mg/kg/24h IM/IV divide q8-12h. *P:* 15-40 μg/ml; *T:* <2 μg/ml.

<u>netilmicin</u> [Netromycin] (Vials 150 mg/1.5cc) *ADULTS* 4-6.5 mg/kg/24h divide q8-12h. *P:* 4-12 μg/ml; *T:* <4 μg/ml. Weight based on lean body mass.

<u>streptomycin sulfate</u> (Vials 1 gram/2.5cc) *ADULTS* 1-2g IM divide q6-12h; *PEDS* 20-40 mg/kg/24h divide q6-12h

<u>tobramycin</u> [Nebcin] (Vials 10 mg/cc, 40 mg/cc) 1-1.66 mg/kg IV/IM q8h (max 5 mg/kg/24h). Infuse over 20-60 mins. *P:* <12 μg/ml; *T:* <2 μg/ml.

β -LACTAMS, MISCELLANEOUS (C – carbapenem class; M – monobactam class)

<u>loracarbef</u> [Lorabid] (Pulvules 200 mg; Susp 100, 200 mg/5cc) *ADULTS use* 200-400 mg PO q12h; *6 mos-12 yrs* use 15-30 mg/kg/24h PO divided q12h. C

<u>aztreonam</u> [Azactam] (Vials 500 mg, 1 & 2 gm) 9 mos – 16 yrs use 30 mg/kg IV/IM q6-8 hours; ★ > 16 yrs- 500 mg - 2 gm IVPB q6-12h, type of infection dependent. M

<u>meropenem</u> [Merrem IV] IVPB .5-1gm Q8h. C

CEPHALOSPORINS
FIRST GENERATION

<u>cefadroxil</u> [Duricef] (Tab 1gm; Cap 500 mg; Susp 125, 250, 500 mg/5cc) *ADULTS use* 1-2gm PO divided QD or BID. *PEDS* use 30 mg/kg/24h divided q12h

<u>cefazolin</u> [Kefzol, Ancef] (Vial 500 mg & 1 gm) *ADULTS use* 250 mg to 1.5 grams IV/IM q6h/q8h/q12h depending on type, site, and severity of infection. *PEDS* use 25-100 mg/kg/24h divided q6h or q8h

<u>cephalexin</u> [Keflex, Keftab] (Tab 250, 500 mg; Susp 125, 250 mg/5cc) *ADULTS use* 1-4 gm/24h divided q6h *PEDS* use 25-50 mg/kg/24h q6h. May divide q12h for strep pharyngitis, skin infections, & uncomplicated UTI.

<u>cephalothin</u> [Keflin] 500 mg - 2 gm IV/IM q6h to q4h

<u>cephapirin</u> [Cefadyl] 500 mg - 2 gm IV/IM q6h to q4h

<u>cephradine</u> [Velosef] 500 mg - 2 gm IV/IM q6h to q4h; 250 mg - 500 mg PO q6h

SECOND GENERATION

<u>cefaclor</u> [Ceclor] (Tab 250, 500 mg; Susp 125, 187, 250, 375 mg) *ADULTS use* 250-500 mg PO q8h; *PEDS* use 20 (pharyngitis) - 40 (otitis media) mg/kg/24h PO divided BID/TID

<u>cefamandole</u> [Mandol] (Vials .5 mg,1,2 g) 500 mg-2 g IM/IV q4h-8h; *PEDS* 50-100 mg/kg/24h IM/IV divide q4-8h

<u>cefmetazole</u> [Zefazone] (Vials 1, 2 gm) 2 gm IV q6h-12h

<u>cefonicid</u> [Monocid] (Vials 500 mg, 1 gm) 1 gm IV/IM q24h

<u>cefotetan</u> [Cefotan] (Vials 1, 2 gm) 1-2 gm IM/IV q12h

<u>cefoxitin</u> [Mefoxin] (Vials 1, 2 gm) 1-2 gm IM/IV q6h-8h

<u>cefuroxime</u> [Zinacef] (Vials 750 mg, 1.5 gm) 750 mg-1.5 gm IM/IV q8h; *PEDS >3mos* use 50-100 mg/kg/24h IM/IV divided q6-8h

<u>cefuroxime</u> [Ceftin] (Susp 125 & 250mg/5ml; Tab 125, 250, 500 mg) *ADULTS- Acute bronchitis* 250-500 mg BID X 5 days; *Gonorrhea* 1 g single dose; *Lyme disease* 500 mg BID X 20 days; *PEDS 3mos–12yrs* use 20 (*pharyngitis/tonsillitis*) – 30 (*Otitis media, maxillary sinusitis, impetigo*) mg/kg/D divided BID. MAX 1 g/D

THIRD GENERATION

<u>cefdinir</u> [Omnicef] (Cap 300 mg; Susp 125 mg/5 ml) 600 mg daily divided BID or QD; skin inf and CAP BID dosing recommended. ★

<u>cefepime hydrochloride</u> [Maxipime] (Vials 0.5, 1, 2 g) IV .5-2 g q12h over 30 min; IM 0.5-1 g q12h

<u>cefixime</u> [Suprax] (Tab 200, 400 mg; Susp 100 mg/5cc) *ADULTS use* 400 mg PO QD or 200 mg PO BID; *PEDS* use 8 mg/kg/24h PO dosed QD or BID

<u>cefprozil</u> [Cefzil] (Tab 250, 500 mg; Susp 125, 250 mg/5cc) *ADULTS use* 250-500 mg q12h; *6mos-12 yrs* use 7.5-15 mg/kg PO q12h

<u>cefpodoxime</u> [Vantin] (Tab 100, 200 mg; Susp 50, 100 mg/5cc) *ADULTS use* 100-400 mg PO q12h; *PEDS* use 10 mg/kg/24h PO divided q12h

<u>cefoperazone</u> [Cefobid] (Vials 1, 2 gm) 2 - 4 gm IV/IM QD divided into q12h doses

<u>cefotaxime</u> [Claforan] (Vials 500 mg, 1, 2 gm) 1 - 2 gm IV/IM q4-12h depending on type of infection

<u>ceftazidime</u> [Fortaz, Tazidime, Tazicef] (Vials 500 mg, 1, 2 gm) 1 gm IV/IM q8-12h

<u>ceftibuten</u> [Cedax] (Cap 400 mg; Susp 90, 180 mg/5ml) *Peds* 9 mg/kg PO MAX 400 mg/D; *Adults* 400 mg QD.

ceftizoxime [Cefizox] ADULTS use 1 - 2 gm IV/IM q8-12h; PEDS use 50 mg/kg/dose IV/IM q6-8h
ceftriaxone [Rocephin] (Vials 250, 500 mg, 1, 2 gm) 1-2 gm IV/IM QD; Uncomplicated gonorrhea use 250 mg IM single dose; PEDS use 50-75 mg/kg IV/IM QD; Meningitis use 100 mg/kg IV/IM QD (do not exceed 4 gm); Otitis media 50 mg/kg (up to 1 g) IM single dose

FLUOROQUINOLONES
alatrofloxacin [Trovan I.V.] withdrawn from the market in 1999 ★
ciprofloxacin [Cipro] (Sol 250 mg/5 ml, 500 mg/5 ml; Tab 250, 500, 750 mg; Vials 200, 400 mg) ADULTS use 250-750 mg PO q12h, OR, 200-400 mg IVPB q12h. immunocompromised - 400mg IVPB q 8h ★ (not recommended for use if <18yrs old)
enoxacin [Penetrex] (Tab 200, 400 mg) 200-400 mg PO q12h, or 400 mg PO single dose for uncomplicated GC
grepafloxacin [Raxar] (Tab 200 mg) 400-600 mg PO QD; 400 mg single dose for uncomplicated GC
levofloxacin [Levaquin] (Tabs 250, 500 mg; Premix inj. 250 mg in 50cc,500 mg in 100cc D5)PO/IV 250-500 mg q24°, *uncomplicated UTI's use* 1 tab QD X 3 days ★
lomefloxacin [Maxaquin] (Tab 400 mg) 400 mg PO QD, *uncomplicated UTI's use* 1 tab QD X 3 days
norfloxacin [Noroxin] (Tab 400 mg) 400 mg PO q12h, or 800 mg PO single dose for uncomplicated GC
ofloxacin [Floxin] (Tab 200, 300, 400 mg; Vials 200, 400 mg) 200-400 mg PO/IV q12h, or 400 mg PO/IV single dose for uncomplicated GC, PID (Chlamydia, gonorrhea) 400 mg BID for 10-14 days
sparfloxacin [Zagam] (Tabs 200 mg) 400 mg PO day one, then 200 mg PO q24°
trovafloxacin [Trovan] withdrawn from the market in 1999 ★

PENICILLINS
Natural
Bicilin C-R [Pen G benzathine + Pen G procaine mix] (equal mix vials of 0.3, 0.6, 1.2, & 2.4 million units/cc, OR 900,000/300,000 unit mix vials) ADULTS >60 lbs use 2.4 million units IM; PEDS 30-60 lbs use 0.9-1.2 million units IM; PEDS <30 lbs use 0.6 million units IM
penicillin G 12-24 million units/24h IVPB divided q4-6h
penicillin G benzathine [Bicillin L-A] ADULTS 1.2 million units deep IM; >27kg (60 lbs) 900,000-1,200,000 units deep IM; <27kg (60 lbs) 300,000-600,000 units deep IM, neonates 50,000 u/kg IM
penicillin G potassium [Pfizerpen] 0.5-80 million units IM/IV QD; (age & type of infection dependent)
penicillin G procaine [Pfizerpen-AS, Wycillin] 0.6-1.0 million units IM QD
penicillin V potassium [Pen Vee K, Ledercillin VK] (250, 500 tablets; 400,000 units = 250 mg) 125-500 mg PO QID; PEDS use 25-50 mg/kg/24h divided q6-8h. (acid stable)

Penicillinase-resistant
cloxacillin [Cloxapen, Tegopen] (Cap 250, 500 mg; Susp 125 mg/5cc) ADULTS use 250 mg - 1 gm PO q6h; PEDS use 100 mg/kg/24h divided q6h
dicloxacillin [Dycill, Dynapen, Pathocil] (Cap 125, 250, 500 mg; Susp 62.5 mg/5cc) ADULTS use 125-250 mg PO q6h; PEDS use 12.5-25 mg/kg/24h divided q6h
methicillin [Staphcillin] (Vials 1, 4, 6 gm) ADULTS use 4-12 gm/24h IM/IV divided q4-6h; PEDS use 100-300 mg/kg/24h IM/IV divided q4-6h; INFANTS - dosage varies
nafcillin [Nafcil, Unipen, Nallpen] (Vials 500 mg, 1, 1.5, 2, 4 gm; 250 mg capsules; 500 mg tablets; Susp 250 mg/5cc) ADULTS use 500 mg-1gm IV/IM q4-6h, OR, 250-500 mg PO q4-6h; PEDS use 25 mg/kg IV/IM BID, OR, 50 mg/kg/24h PO divided QID
oxacillin [Bactocill, Prostaphlin] (Vials 250, 500 mg, 1, 2, 4 gm; Cap 250, 500 mg; Sol 250 mg/5cc) PARENTERAL: ADULTS use 250 mg-1g IV/IM q4-6h; PEDS(<40lbs) use 50-100 mg/kg/24h IV/IM divided q6h. ORAL: ADULTS use 500 mg-1g PO q4-6h; PEDS(<40lbs) use 50-100 mg/kg/24h PO divided q6h

Ampicillins
amoxicillin [Amoxil] (Chew 125, 250 mg; Cap 250, 500 mg; Susp 50, 125, 250 mg/5cc) ADULTS use 250-500 mg PO q8h; PEDS use 20-40 mg/kg/24h PO divided q8h
ampicillin [Omnipen, Principen] (Vials 125, 250, 500 mg, 1, 2gm; Cap 250, 500, 875 mg; Susp 100, 125, 250, 500 mg/5cc) ADULTS: 1-12 g/24h IV/IM/PO divided q6-12h; PEDS 50-200 mg/kg/24h IV/IM/PO divided q6h
Augmentin [ampicillin/clavulanate] (Tab 250, 500, 875 mg; Chw 125, 200, 250, 400 mg; Susp 125, 200, 250, 400 mg/5cc) ADULTS (>40kg) use 250-500 mg tid or 500-875 mg PO bid; PEDS see Pediatrics
bacampicillin [Spectrobid] (Tab 400 mg; 125 mg/5cc suspension) ADULTS use 400-800 mg PO q12h; PEDS use 25-50 mg/kg/24h PO q12h
Unasyn [ampicillin/sulbactam] (Vial 1.5, 3gm) 1.5-3 gm IVPB q6-8h

Extended Spectrum Penicillins
carbenicillin [Geocillin] (Tab 382 mg) 1-2 tabs PO QID
mezlocillin [Mezlin] (Vials 1, 2, 3, 4 gm) 1.5-4 gm IVPB q4-8h, OR, 100-350 mg/kg/24h divided q4-8h
piperacillin [Pipracil] (Vials 2, 3, 4 gm) 3-4 gm IVPB q4-6h, OR, 200-500 mg/kg/24h divided q4-6h

ticarcillin [Ticar] (Vials 1, 3, 6 gm) 1-4 gm IV/IM q3-6h, OR, 200-300 mg/kg/24h divided q3-6h

Timentin [ticarcillin/clavulanate] (Vials 3.1 gm) *ADULTS* 3.1 gm IV q4-6h; *PEDS* >3 mo: < 60 kg mild-moderate infection 200 mg/kg/d dosed q6h, severe infection 300 mg/kg/d dosed q4h; > 60 kg mild-moderate infection 3.1 g q6h, severe infection 3.1 g q4h

Zosyn [piperacillin/tazobactam] (Vials 2g/.25g, 3g/.375g, 4g/.5g) ADULTS use 3.375g IVPB q6h

MACROLIDES

azithromycin [Zithromax] (Tab 250 mg, Z-PAKS of 6 250 mg, 600 mg; Susp 100, 200 mg/5ml, Packets 1gm; Inj 500 mg/vial) 500 mg PO day 1, then 250 mg PO QD X 4 days; *Community-acquired pneumonia* 500 mg IV (over >60mins) QD X 2days follow with 500 mg PO QD X 5-8 more days; *PID* 500 mg IV QD X 2days follow with 250 mg PO QD X 5days; *Peds:* 10 mg/kg day 1, then 5 mg/kg QD X 4days; *Pharyngitis* 12 mg/kg QD X 5 days. (1 g single dose for chancroid or non-gonococcal urethritis & cervicitis due to chlamydia; 2g single dose for gonorrhea)

clarithromycin [Biaxin](Susp 125 &250 mg/5ml;Tab 250,500 mg) Peds 7.5 mg/kg BID; Adults 250-500 mg q12h

dirithromycin [Dynabac] (Tab 250 mg) PO >12 yr old- 500 mg QD X 7D for *bronchitis, uncomplicated skin*; X 14d for *Pneumonia*

erythromycin base [ERYC(250 mg), E-mycin(250, 333 mg), PCE(333, 500 mg), Ery-Tab(250, 333, 500 mg)] 250 mg PO q6h, or 333 mg PO q8h, or 500 mg PO q12h

erythromycin estolate [Ilosone] (Tab 250, 500 mg; Susp 125, 250 mg/5cc) ADULTS use 250 mg PO q6h; PEDS use 30-50 mg/kg/24h PO divided q6 or 12h

erythromycin ethylsuccinate [EES, EryPed] (Tab 400 mg; Susp 200, 400 mg/5cc; Drp 100 mg/5cc) ADULTS use 400 mg PO q6h; PEDS use 30-50 mg/kg/24h PO divided q6, 8, or 12h

erythromycin lactobionate (Vial 500 mg, 1 gm) 15-20 mg/kg/24h IV divided q6h (4 grams/24h max)

erythromycin stearate [Erythrocin stearate] (Tab 250 mg) 250 mg q6h or 500 mg q12h

Pediazole [200 mg erythromycin ethylsuccinate + 600 mg sulfisoxazole per 5cc] 50 mg/kg/24h based on erythromycin component, OR 150 mg/kg/24h based on sulfa component, divided equally q6 or 8h

troleandomycin [TAO] (Cap 250 mg) ADULTS use 250-500 mg PO QID; PEDS use 125-250 mg PO q6h

SULFONAMIDES

trimethoprim/sulfamethoxazole [Bactrim, Septra] (Tab 80/200 mg; DS 160/800 mg; Susp 40/200 mg /5cc) 5 mg/kg IV q6h (based on TMX); 1 DS tab OR 2 single strength tablets OR 4 tsps susp PO BID; PEDS use 8 mg/kg/24h TMX & 40 mg/kg/24h SMX PO divided BID

Pediazole — see under macrolides

sulfadiazine [generic] (Tab 500 mg) 2-4g QD in 3-6 divided doses

sulfamethizole [Thiosulfil Forte] (Tab 500 mg) 0.5-1g PO 3-4 times daily

sulfamethoxazole [Gantanol] (Tab 500 mg; Susp 500 mg/5ml) PO 1000 mg TID

sulfisoxazole [Gantrisin] (Tab 500 mg; syrup-chocolate 500 mg/5cc; ped susp-raspberry 500 mg/5cc) ADULTS use initial dose of 2-4 gm followed by a maintenance dose of 4-8 gm/24h divided q4-6h; PEDS use inititally ½ of 24h dose, followed by maintenance dose of 150 mg/kg/24h divided q4-6h

ANTIMYCOTICS, SYSTEMIC

amphotericin B [Fungizone IV] (50 mg/vial) Test Dose = 1 mg slowly IV; Begin with 0.25 mg/kg/24h IV, then gradually increase to a total daily dose of 1-1.5 mg/kg

amphotericin B [Ambisome] (50 mg/vial as liposome) IV over ≥2 hours; *Age ≥1 month-* Empirical therapy use 3 mg/kg/day; *Systemic fungal infections* use 3-5 mg/kg/day

fluconazole [Diflucan] (Tab 50, 100, 150, 200 mg; Sol 10mg/ml, 40mg/ml; Vials 200 mg/100cc, 400 mg/200cc) Initial dose 200 mg PO/IV QD, followed by 100-200 mg PO/IVPB QD

flucytosine [Ancobon] (Cap 250, 500 mg) 50-150 mg/kg/24h PO divided q6h

griseofulvin [Fulvicin U/F (microsize), Fulvicin P/G (ultramicrosize)] [Tab microsize-250, 500 mg; Cap 125, 250 mg; Susp 125 mg/5cc] (Tab ultramicrosize-125, 165,250, 300 mg) 500 mg-1gm (microsize) or 330-750 mg (ultramicrosize) PO QD

itraconazole [Sporanox] (Cap 100 mg, Sol 10 mg/ml) 200-400 mg PO QD, if daily dose >200 mg, divide BID; Oropharyngeal candidiasis 200 mg QD by swish & swallow 10 ml at a time, Oropharyngeal candidiasis refractory to fluconazole use 100 mg BID. Onychomycosis: toenails 200 mg QD X 12 consecutive wks; fingernails 200 mg BID X 1 wk, then skip 3 wks and repeat.

ketoconazole [Nizoral] (Tab 200 mg) ADULTS use 200-400 mg PO QD; PEDS use 3.3-6.6 mg/kg/24h PO QD

miconazole [Monistat] (10 mg/cc) 200-3600 mg/24h IVPB may be divided q8h; dosage varies widely

nystatin, oral [Mycostatin] (Tab 500,000U, Pastilles 200000U, Susp 100000U/ml in 60ml with dropper) *Adults* 500,000-1,000,000U PO TID, 1-2 pastilles dissolved in mouth 4-5 times/D, 4-6ml QID; *Infants* 2ml QID

terbinafine [Lamisil] (Tab 250 mg; Cream and Sol – see Dermatology section) Onychomycosis: Fingernail – PO 250 mg/day for 6 weeks; Toenail – PO 250 mg/day for 12 weeks

TETRACYCLINES

<u>tetracycline</u> (Cap 100, 200, 250, 500 mg; Susp 125 mg/5cc; Inj 100, 250, 500 mg) 250-500 mg PO BID-QID, OR, 250-500 mg IV/IM q12h

<u>demeclocycline</u> [Declomycin] (Cap 150 mg; Tab 150 mg, 300 mg) 150 mg PO QID, OR, 300 mg PO BID

<u>doxycycline</u> [Vibramycin] (Tab/Cap 50, 100 mg; Susp 25 mg/5cc; Syp 50 mg/5cc; Inj 100, 200 mg) 200 mg PO/IVPB day one, followed by 100 mg/24h PO/IVPB QD or divided q12h. Do not give to children<8yrs old or inject IM/SC

<u>methacycline</u> [Rondomycin] (Cap 150, 300 mg) 600 mg/24h PO divided BID or QID

<u>minocycline</u> [Minocin] (Tab/Cap 50, 100 mg; Susp 50 mg/5cc; Inj 100 mg) 200 mg PO/IVPB first dose, followed by 200 mg/24h PO/IVPB divided q6-12h

<u>oxytetracycline</u> [Terramycin] (Cap 250 mg; Inj 50, 125 mg) Oral dosing same as tetracycline; 250 mg IVPB q24h, OR, 300 mg IVPB divided q8-12h

URINARY ANTI-INFECTIVES

<u>cinoxacin</u> [Cinobac] (Cap 250, 500 mg) 1g/day divided BID or QID

<u>methenamine hippurate</u> [Hiprex, Urex] (Tab 1g) 0.5-1g PO BID

<u>methenamine mandelate</u> [Mandelamine] (Tab 0.5, 1g; Susp 25 mg/5cc; Forte 50 mg/5cc) ADULTS use 1g PO QID; PEDS(6-12yrs) use 0.5g PO QID, (<6yrs) use 25mr/14kg PO QID

<u>methylene blue</u> [Urolene blue] (Tab 55, 65 mg) 55-130 mg PO TID after meals with full glass of water

<u>nalidixic acid</u> [NegGram] (Cap 250, 500mg,1g; Susp 250mg/5cc) *Adults* 1g QID; *Peds* 55mg/kg/day divided QID

<u>nitrofurantoin macrocrytals</u> [Macrodantin] (Cap 25, 50, 100 mg) ADULTS use 50-100 mg PO QID AC & HS; PEDS use 5-7 mg/kg/24h divided QID

MISCELLANEOUS ANTIBIOTICS

<u>chloramphenicol</u> [Chloromycetin] (Cap 250 mg, Susp 150 mg/5cc, Inj 100 mg/cc) ADULTS & PEDS use 50-100 mg/kg/24h divided q6h

<u>clindamycin</u> [Cleocin] (Cap 75, 150, 300 mg; Sol 75 mg/5cc; Vial 150 mg/cc) 150-300 mg PO q6h; 600-1200 mg/24h IVPB divided q6-12h

<u>fosfomycin</u> [Monurol] (granules 3g) Mix 1 sachet in 3-4oz water, drink immediately. *uncomplicated UTI*

<u>furazolidone</u> [Furoxone] (Tab 100 mg; Liq50 mg/15cc) ADULTS - 100 mg QID; PEDS(≥5yrs) - 25-50 mg QID.

<u>lincomycin</u> [Lincocin] (Cap 500 mg; Inj 300 mg/ml) ADULTS use 500 mg PO q8h, OR, 600 mg IM q12-24h, OR, 600 mg/12 g IVPB q8-12h; PEDS use 30-60 mg/kg/24h PO divided with 6-8h

<u>metronidazole</u> [Flagyl] (Cap 375 mg; Tab 250, 500, ER 750 mg; Inj 500 mg) Load q15 mg/kg IVPB, follow with 7.5 mg/kg IVPB q6h OR, 7.5 mg/kg PO q6h; Flagyl ER 750 mg tabs QD for bacterial vaginosis

<u>Primaxin</u> [imipenem/cilastatin] (250 mg/250 mg, 500 mg/500 mg, 750 mg/750 mg) 250 mg-1gm IVPB/IM q6-8h; Peds - mild-to-moderate infections: 10 to 15 mg/kg IVPB q6h

<u>spectinomycin</u> [Trobicin](Vial 100 mg,2,4gm)2gm IM single dose for gonorrhea, 4gm IM if resistance is prevalent

<u>trimethoprim</u> [Proloprim, Trimpex] (100, 200 mg Tabs) 200 mg PO QD, or 100 mg PO BID

<u>vancomycin</u> [Vancocil] (Pulvules 125, 250 mg; Sol 250 mg/5cc, 500 mg/5cc) ADULTS use 500 mg-2g/24h divided q6h, OR, 500 mg IVPB 6h or 1g IVPB q12h; *PEDS use* 40 mg/kg/24h PO q6-8h or 10 mg/kg/dose IVPB q6h

ANTITUBERCULOUS DRUGS

<u>capreomycin</u> [Capastat Sulfate] (Inj 1g/10cc) 1g IM daily

<u>cycloserine</u> [Seromycin Pulvules] (250 mg) 0.5-1g PO QD in divided doses (monitor blood levels <30 µg/ml)

<u>ethambutol</u> [Myambutol] (Tab 100, 400 mg) 15 mg/kg PO QD

<u>ethionamide</u> [Trecator-SC] (Tab 250 mg) ADULTS use 0.5-1g/24h in divided doses; PEDS use 15-20 mg/kg/24h

<u>isoniazid</u> [Laniazid] (Tab 100, 300 mg; Syp 50 mg/5cc; Inj 100 mg/cc) ADULTS use 5 mg/kg/24h PO/IM QD; PEDS use 10-20 mg/kg/24h PO/IM QD

<u>p-aminosalicylic acid</u> [Sodium P.A.S.] (Tab 0.5g) ADULTS use 14-16g/kg/24h in 2-3 divided doses; PEDS use 275-420 mg/kg/24h in 3-4 divided doses

<u>pyrazinamide</u> (Tab 500 mg) 15-30 mg/kg PO QD, do not exceed 2g/day

<u>rifabutin</u> [Mycobutin] (Cap 150 mg) 300 mg PO QD

<u>rifampin</u> [Rifadin] (Cap 150, 300 mg; Inj 600 mg) 600 mg PO/IV QD for TB; 600 mg BID for 2 days for meningococcal carriers (MC); *PEDS use* 10-20 mg/kg PO/IV QD not to exceed 600 mg/day for TB; BID for MC

<u>rifapentine</u> [Priftin] TB drug (Tab 150 mg) PO 600 mg twice weekly for 2 months

<u>Rifater</u> [rifampin 120 mg, isoniazid 50 mg, pyrazinamide 300 mg] Tab. Dosage varies based on patient weight

INH Preventative Therapy (54-88% effective against developing active TB for 20yrs) 6 groups without age limit:
- HIV+ (Active disease risk is 10%/YR & is 113X increased in HIV+ pts.. & 170X ↑ in AIDS Pts..)
- Household members of persons with recently diagnosed tuberculous disease (↑risk of 2-4%/yr)
- Newly infected persons as presenting with a + Tuberculin skin test within past 2 yrs. (↑ risk of 3.3% 1st yr)
- Previous TB not treated with adequate chemotherapy (such as INH, rifampin, etc.)
- (+) tuberculin reactors with CXR consistent with non-progressive tuberculous disease (↑risk of 0.5-5%/yr)
- (+) tuberculin reactors with specific underlying predisposing conditions, such as: IV drug use, DM, silicosis, steroid dependent (>15 mg prednisone/day), immunosuppressive , hematologic diseases (Hodgkins, leukemia, etc.), ESRD, gastrectomy, clinical cond. with substantial rapid wt. loss or chronic malnutrition

Tuberculin skin test (TBST) interpretation:[MMWR 43 (RR13:59,1994)]
≥5mm is + in the following: HIV+ or risk factors, recent close contacts, CXR consistent with healed TB.
≥10mm is + in the following: foreign-born in countries of high prevalence, IV drug users, low income populations, nursing home residents, pts.. with medical cond. which increasess risk (see above).
≥15mm is + in all others.
- 2-step TBST (for use in persons regularly tested, e.g., health-care workers): If 1st TBST is reactive yet <10mm, repeat 5 TU in 1 week, if then ≥10mm test is +, but not a recent conversion.
- BCG vaccination may produce a reactive TBST, yet, if ≥10mm in an adult who was vaccinated as a child & from a country with a high prevalence of TB should be considered infected.

LEPROSTATICS
dapsone (Tab 25, 100 mg) 50-100 mg PO QD
clofazimine [Lamprene] (Cap 50, 100 mg) 100-200 mg PO QD

AMEBICIDES
Emetine (Inj 65 mg/cc) 1 mg/kg/24h deep SC/IM QD
Iodoquinol [Yodoxin] (Tab 210, 650 mg) ADULTS use 650 mg PO TID; PEDS - 40 mg/kg/24h in 3 divided doses
metronidazole [Flagyl] (Cap 375 mg; Tab 250, 500 mg) 250-750 mg PO TID
paromomycin [Humatin] (Cap 250 mg) 25-35 mg/kg/24h in 3 divided doses daily

ANTIHELMINTICS
albendazole [Albenza] (Tab 200 mg) ≥60kg use 400 mg PO BID; <60kg use 15 mg/kg/day. *hydatid disease & neurocysticercosis*
diethylcarbamazine [Hetrazan] (Tab 50 mg) *filariasis, onchocerciasis & loiasis* 2 mg/kg TID; *ascariasis* 13 mg/kg QD X 7 days; compassionate use only – free of charge from Wyeth-Ayerst Labs
ivermectin [Stromectol] (Tab 6 mg) Use single PO dose to provide ≈0.2 mg/kg (*Strongyloidiasis*) or ≈0.15 mg/kg (*Onchocerciasis*)
mebendazole [Vermox] (Chw 100 mg) 1 tab morning & evening X 3 days; *Enterobiasis* 1 tab single dose
oxamniquine [Vansil] (Cap 250 mg) ADULTS - 12-15 mg/kg single dose; (<30kg) - 10 mg/kg BID
praziquantel [Biltricide] (Tab 600 mg) 20-25 mg/kg TID X 1 day
pyrantel [Antiminth-50 mg/cc suspension; Reese's pinworm(OTC)-50 mg/cc liquid] 11 mg/kg single dose
thiabendazole [Mintezol] (Chw 500 mg; Susp 500 mg/5cc) 22 mg/kg/dose BID

ANTIPROTOZOALS
atovaquone [Mepron] (Tab 250 mg) 750 mg PO TID
eflornithine [Ornidyl] (Inj 200 mg/ml) 100 mg/kg/dose iv q6hby IV infusion for 14 days

ANTIMALARIALS
chloroquine HCl [Aralen HCl] (Inj 50 mg/cc) 4-5cc IM initially, repeat in 6h if necessary.
chloroquine phosphate [Aralen phosphate] (Tab 250, 500 mg) dosage varies
halofantrine [Halfan] (Tab 250 mg) PO 500 mg every 6 hours for 3 doses, take on an empty stomach at least 1 hour before or 2 hours after food, repeat course 7 days after the first
hydroxychloroquine sulfate [Plaquenil sulfate] (Tab 200 mg) 2 tablets weekly (prophylaxis)
mefloquine HCl [Lariam] (Tab 250 mg) For *malaria treatment* use 5 tablets PO as single dose; For malaria prophylaxis use 250 mg once weekly X 4 weeks, then 250 mg every other week
primaquine phosphate (Tab 26.3 mg) 1 tab QD X 14 days
pyrimethamine [Daraprim] (Tab 25 mg) dosage varies
sulfadoxine/pyrimethamine [Fansidar] (Tab 500 mg/25 mg) dosage varies

ANTIVIRAL AGENTS

<u>Avonex</u> [Interferon beta-1a] (33mcg/vial) >18yoa use 30mcg IM once weekly. *multiple sclerosis*

<u>acyclovir</u> [Zovirax] (Tab 400, 800 mg; Cap 200 mg; Susp 200 mg/5cc) *Initial genital herpes* 200 mg PO q4h; *Chronic suppression* 400 mg PO BID; *Herpes zoster* 800 mg q4h. For IV see under AIDS section

<u>amantadine</u> [Symmetrel] (Cap 100 mg; Syp 50 mg/5cc) ADULTS - 200 mg PO QD; PEDS (9-12yrs) - 100 mg BID; (1-9yrs) 2-4 mg/lb/24h QD or divided BID

<u>famciclovir</u> [Famvir] (Tab 125, 250, 500 mg) *Herpes Zoster* - 500 mg q8h X 7D; *genital herpes* 125 mg BID X 5 D; *Suppression recurrent genital herpes (≥6 episodes/yr)* 250 mg BID, then reevaluate after 1 year; adjust for CrCl

<u>interferon alfa-2b</u> [Intron A] (3, 5, 10, 18, 25 million IU/vials) *>18yoa Genital warts* use 1 million IU injected intralesionally/lesion 3 times weekly; Chronic Hepatitis B patients > 1 years of age

<u>interferon alfa-2a</u> [Roferon-A] (3, 6, 9, 18, 36 million IU/vial) *>18yoa* use 3-6 million IU SC or IM 3 times weekly for 12 months. Chronic Hepatitis C

<u>interferon alfa-n1</u> [Wellferon] (Sol 3 MU/ml) 3 MU SC or IM 3 times per week for 48 weeks (12 months). *Hepatitis C*★

<u>interferon alfacon-1</u> [Infergen] (9, 15 mcg/vial) *>18yoa* use 9 mcg SC 3 times weekly at least 48 hrs apart for 24 weeks; For unresponsive or relapsed may use 15 mcg SC 3 times weekly for 24 wks. Chronic Hepatitis C

<u>oseltamivir</u> [Tamiflu] (Cap 75mg) PO ≥ 18 years of age is 1 Cap twice daily for 5 days. Begin treatment within the first 2 days of symptoms. New neuraminidase inhibitor -treatment of uncomplicated acute illness due to influenza virus.★

<u>Rebetron</u> [interferon alfa-2b 3 million IU vials/Ribavirin 200 mg] Chronic Hepatitis C: <75 kg- Ribavirin 400 mg PO AM and 600 mg PM; >75 kg- 600 mg BID; interferon alfa 3 million IU SC 3 times a week

<u>ribavirin</u> [Virazole] (20 mg/ml after reconstituted) aerosol use only for severe lower respiratory tract RSV infections. Treatment 12-18° a day for 3-7 days

<u>rimantadine</u> [Flumadine] (Tab 100 mg; Syp 50 mg/5cc) ADULTS - 100 mg PO BID; PEDS - 5 mg/kg PO QD

<u>ritonavir</u> [Norvir] (Tab 100 mg, Oral Sol 600 mg/7.5ml)PO with meals 600 mg BID

<u>valacyclovir</u> [Valtrex] (Cap 500 mg) *Herpes Zoster* - 2 caps (1g) TID X 7 days; *initial episode of genital herpes* 1 g BID X 5 days; *Treatment of recurrent genital herpes* 500 mg q12 hrs X 5 days; *Suppression of recurrent genital herpes* 1 g QD, alternate dose (≤9 episodes/yr) 500 mg QD, reevaluate in 1 yr

<u>vidarabine</u> [Vira-A] (20 mg/cc injectable) 10-15 mg/kg/24h IV

<u>zanamivir</u> [Relenza] (diskhaler device 5mg/inh) ≥ 12 years of age is 2 inh twice daily for 5 days. Begin treatment within the first 2 days of symptoms. New neuraminidase inhibitor -treatment of uncomplicated acute illness due to influenza virus.★

Infectious Disease Notes:

FORMULAS

$$\text{Creatinine Clearance} = \frac{(140 - \text{Age})(\text{weight in kg})}{(72)(\text{serum creatinine})} \times (0.85 \text{ for women})[\text{normal} = 75 - 160\text{ml/min}]$$

$$\text{Clearance} = \frac{U \times V}{P} \quad [\text{inulin is more accurate, although creatinine usually used}]$$

$$\text{GFR} = 125 \text{ ml/min}$$

$$\text{Renal blood flow} = 1200 \text{ ml/min} = \frac{RPF}{1 - HCT}$$

$$\text{Renal plasma flow} = 1/2 \text{ renal blood flow} = 600 \text{ ml/min}$$

$$\text{Plasma osmolality} = 2(Na^+) + \frac{\text{glucose}}{18} + \frac{BUN}{2.8} + \frac{\text{ethanol}}{4.6} \quad [\text{normal} = 275 - 295 \text{ mosm}]$$

Total Body Water (TBW) (L) men = $0.6 \times$ lean body weight in kg; women = $0.5 \times$ weight in kg

$$\text{Desired Total Body Water (L)} = \frac{PNa^+ \times TBW}{\text{Normal serum } Na^+}$$

$$Na^+ \text{deficit (mEq)} = \left[(TBW)(140 - PNa+)\right]$$

$$\text{Water deficit (L)} = TBW \times \left(\frac{\text{Plasma } Na^+}{140} - 1\right)$$

$$FENa^+ = \frac{Na^+ \text{ excreted}}{Na^+ \text{ filtered}} \times 100 = \frac{(UNa^+)(PCr)}{(PNa^+)(UCr)} \times 100$$

$$\text{Renal failure index (RFI)} = \frac{(UNa^+)(PCr)}{(UCr)}$$

ELECTROLYTES

HYPONATREMIA

"Disorder of water balance". Serum Sodium < 135 meq/L.

HYPERTONIC HYPONATREMIA

DX: Increased Serum Osmolality > 290 mosm/kg H_2O and low sodium
DDX: Hyperglycemia: $Na^+ \downarrow$ 1.6 meq/L for each 100 mg/dl rise in glucose
    Hypertonic Infusions: Glucose - $Na^+ \downarrow$ 1.6 meq/L for each 100 mg/dl rise in glucose
                       Mannitol - $Na^+ \downarrow$ 1.6 meq/L for each 100 mg/dl rise in mannitol
                       Glycine - $Na^+ \downarrow$ 3.8 meq/L for each 100 mg/dl rise in glycine
TREATMENT: Correct volume deficit, Insulin to slowly decrease glucose, Hypotonic saline to correct free water deficit. COMPLICATIONS: Hypoglycemia, cerebral edema

ISOTONIC HYPONATREMIA

DX: Normal measured serum osmolality, $\downarrow$ Sodium
DDX: Hyperlipidemic states: plasma lipid (mg/dl) x 0.002 = the decrease in Na^+ (meq/L)
      Hyperproteinemic states: (measured protein g/dl - 8) x 0.25 = the decrease in Na^+ (meq/L)
TREATMENT: Correct underlying cause. COMPLICATIONS: Related to underlying disease

HYPOTONIC HYPONATREMIA

DX: Decreased measured serum osmolality < 270 mosm/kg H2O, $\downarrow$ Sodium
DDX: <u>Hypovolemic</u>
    Extrarenal: U_{Na+} <20meq/L;GI loss:diarrhea, vomiting; 3rd space loss (e.g. pancreatitis), Burns, Sweating
    Renal: U_{Na+} >20meq/L (cannot reabsorb Na^+); Diuretics, Renal parenchymal disease, Adrenal Failure
    <u>Hypervolemic</u>   Advanced renal failure: Acute renal failure, Chronic renal failure
                                Edematous state: Cirrhosis, CHF, Nephrotic Syndrome, Severe hypoproteinemia
    <u>Isovolemic</u>
    SIADH, Hypothyroidism, $\downarrow K^+$/Diuretic, Psychogenic Polydipsia, Stress, Adrenal Insufficiency, Drugs
TREATMENT: •Hypovolemic: isotonic saline; If Symptomatic - 3% saline (not with edema) correct to 1/3 of TBW [e.g. 80kg pt with serum Na^+ 120 = (.20 x 80kg) x (140 -120)= 320 meq]. Use caution with replacement, by no more than 10 mmol/L (10 meq/L) within 24 h, too rapid correction may cause central pontine myelinolysis. May require use of diuretics to prevent fluid overload. If severe may require ultrafiltration. •Hypervolemic/Isovolemic: restrict free water; • Manage underlying disorders. COMPLICATIONS: Seizures, coma, death, and residual effects

HYPERNATREMIA
H_2O moves from cell to ECF and shrinks cell. Most common cause is $\downarrow H_2O$ intake or H_2O loss > than Na^+ loss
Differential Diagnosis:
- Hypovolemic (volume contraction): H_2O deficit or osmotic diuresis (i.e. Diabetes Mellitus)
- Isovolumic (Diabetes Insipidus)
- Volume overload- excess water and Na^+.

TREATMENT: Fluid replacement, correct **SLOWLY**, too rapid correction can cause cerebral edema. Diuresis if fluid overload

HYPERKALEMIA
Differential Diagnosis: • Acute or chronic renal failure, acidosis, rhabdomyolysis, hemolysis, Iatrogenic (excessive K^+ replacement, K^+ sparing diuretics), false elevation, hemolysis, rhabdomyolysis, Type IV RTA, Adrenal insufficiency, tumor lysis syndrome. Diagnosis: Weakness or paralysis. EKG -peaked T waves, wide QRS, prolonged PR interval.

TREATMENT:
- K^+ 5.5-6.0 meq/L without ECG changes:
  Repeat K^+ level, full set of electrolytes, ECG, check volume status, remove K^+ from IV fluids, check patients medications and hold any that could cause hyperkalemia.
- K^+ >6.0 meq/L with or without ECG changes or 5.5 with ECG changes:
  Admit to telemetry, check electrolytes, BUN, creatinine, ABG, U_{K^+}, U_{Na^+}, U_{Cl}, cortisol levels.
  Administer: Calcium gluconate 1-2 gm slow IV, $NaHCO_3$ 1-2 ampules if acidotic, $D_{10}W$ 125 ml/hr add regular insulin to remain euglycemic and drive K^+ intracellularly. Kayexalate:30-60gm in 30ml sorbitol PO q6h (1gm Kayexalate removes 1 meq K^+) or retention enema (Kayexalate 50 gm, Sorbitol 50 gm, H_2O 200 cc, retained for 30-60 min). Dialysis if needed

HYPOKALEMIA
Differential Diagnosis:
- Intracellular Shift: Alkalosis (H^+ comes out of cell, K^+ moves into cell, $\uparrow$ pH 0.1 = $\downarrow K^+$ of 0.5-0.8) or Administration of insulin/ glucose
- Decreased Intake
- Increased Loss
  Renal: Diuretics, Exogenous steroids, RTA, Primary Hyperaldosteronism, Secondary Hyperaldosteronism (retains Na^+ in exchange for K^+) Cushing's syndrome, Bartter's syndrome, Liddle's syndrome, Penicillins.
  GI Loss: vomiting, diarrhea, fistulas, NG suction, malabsorption, laxative or enema abuse.
Diagnosis: Weakness, paralysis, $\downarrow$ DTR's. ECG –Changes: ST depression, T wave inversion, increased QT interval, Dysrhythmias.

TREATMENT: PO K^+ replacement. Consider IV replacement if symptomatic or severely depleted.
Concentrations > 40 meq/L by central line only.

CALCIUM: Correction for hypoalbuminemia: [(4.5 - measured albumin) x 0.8] + measured Ca^{2+} = corrected Ca^{2+}

ACID BASE
NORMAL VALUES: HCO_3 =24 meq/L, PCO_2=40 mmHg, pH= pK + log(HCO_3 /1.2) = 7.4 = 6.1 + log 24/1.2 = 7.4
ANION GAP=Na^+ - (Cl +HCO_3) Normal = 12-14 mEq/L (accumulation of organic acids)
GOLDEN RULES OF ABGs   • PCO_2 Δ of 10 mmHg = pH Δ of 0.08
                       • HCO_3 Δ of 10 meq/L = pH Δ of 0.15

METABOLIC ACIDOSIS
Differential Diagnosis:
- Renal Disease: Acute or Chronic renal disease, Renal Tubular Acidosis
- Large Acid Loads: Exogenous acidifying agents, Anion Gap Metabolic acidosis (see below).
- GI loss of Bicarbonate: Diarrhea, ureterosigmoidostomy, loss of pancreatic juices (suction or fistula).
Diagnosis: Lethargy, Kussmaul hyperventilation, pH<7.35, HCO_3 <20meq/L, 10meq/L $\uparrow$in HCO_3 = 0.15 $\downarrow$ in pH

ANION GAP ACIDOSIS "MUD PILES"	NON GAP ACIDOSIS "HEART CCU"
Methanol	Hypoaldosteronism
Uremia	Expansion- volume
Diabetic/ethanol/starvation ketoacidosis	Alimentation- TPN
Paraldehyde	RTA Type IV
INH, Nipride, epinephrine, norepinephrine	Trots- Diarrhea
Lactic acidosis	Cholestyramine
Ethylene glycol	Carbonic anhydrase
Salicylates	Ureterosigmoidostomy

RENAL TUBULAR ACIDOSIS

TYPE I: (distal) Decreased distal acidification, ↓ H⁺ secretion. <u>DDX</u>: Albright's or Lightwood's syndrome, hypergammaglobulinemia. <u>DX</u>: Urine pH >5.3. Unable to lower urine pH <5.3 with acid challenge. ↑ Cl⁻, ↓ K⁺. Plasma HCO_3^-: possible < 10 meq/L. Fractional Excretion of HCO_3^- when plasma HCO_3^- >20meq/L is<3%.
TREATMENT: Balance bicarbonate excess with bicarbonate and K⁺ supplements.

TYPE II: (proximal) Hyperchloremic, hypokalemic metabolic acidosis. ↓ proximal HCO_3 reabsorption. <u>DDX</u>: Primary- defective or inhibited carbonic anhydrase (Males only) or Fanconi's Syndrome. <u>DX</u>: Urine pH: >5.3 if above reabsorption threshold, <5.3 if below. Plasma HCO_3^-: possible >10 meq/L. ↑ Cl, ↓ K⁺. Confirm: HCO_3^- infusion to increased plasma pH results in bicarbonaturia. Fractional Excretion of HCO_3 >15-20% when plasma HCO_3^- is > 20meq/L.

TYPE III: Infantile variant of TYPE I.

TYPE IV: Hyperkalemic, hyperchloremic metabolic acidosis. ↓ K⁺ & H⁺ secretion due to defective distal tubule. Common in diabetics; Defective aldosterone production or action. <u>DDX</u>: Addison's, Primary hyporeninemia(Nephrosclerosis, HTN, Diabetic nephropathy), decreased Aldosterone responsiveness (Sickle cell disease, NSAID nephropathy). <u>DX</u>: metabolic acidosis, ↑ K⁺, ↓ Na⁺,↓ Cl⁻.
TREATMENT: Restrict K⁺ & mineralocorticoid administration.

METABOLIC ALKALOSIS
Differential Diagnosis:
↑ HCO_3^- retention: Diuretic therapy, exogenous $NaHCO_3$ administration.
↑ Loss of H⁺: NG suction, Zollinger -Ellison syndrome, emesis, diuretics.
↑ Adrenal steroids: Hyperaldosteronism, exogenous steroids, Cushing's syndrome.
Diagnosis: ↑ CO_2, ↓ Cl , ↓ K⁺, ABG -↑ pH, ↑ PCO_2. Treatment: treat underlying cause.

RESPIRATORY ACIDOSIS: ↓ alveolar ventilation, PCO_2 usually ↑ > 10mmHg. 10mmHg ↑ in PCO_2=.08 ↓ in pH Differential Diagnosis: CNS disorder, neuromuscular disease, hypoventilation, airway obstruction, pulmonary edema, ARDS, pneumothorax. Diagnosis: ABG: Acute: ↑ PCO_2, HCO_3 normal, ↓ PO_2, pH ↓ 0.08; Chronic: HCO_3^- ↑ 3-4 meq/L, ↑ PCO_2, ↓ PO_2, mild ↓ pH. Treatment: Correct cause of ↓ ventilation.

RESPIRATORY ALKALOSIS: ↑ ventilation; Differential Diagnosis: Mechanical ventilation, sepsis, fever, anxiety, pulmonary embolus, poisoning, brainstem or hepatic disease. Diagnosis: Headache, hyperventilation, numbness. ABG- ↑ pH, ↓ PO_2. Treatment: Correct underlying cause.

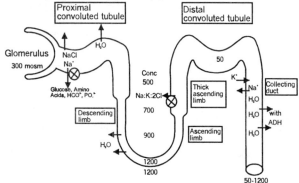

BODY FLUIDS
WATER: 50-60% TBW; ECF 20% TBW [Intravascular 6-7%, Extravascular 12-14%]; ICF 40% TBW.
BLOOD VOLUME: Male 7.2% IBW; Female 7% IBW; Child 8% IBW.
POSTURAL HYPOTENSION: HR ↑ >20 bpm; BP ↓ 10 mmHg = 25% loss

RENAL DYNAMICS
PROXIMAL TUBULE - reabsorbs: Na^+ 60-70%, K^+, sugars, AA's, U.A.,HCO_3 .
DESCENDING LOOP - permeable to H_2O only, fluid becomes hypertonic.
ASCENDING LOOP - Cl pump- Na^+ follows; generates free H_2O.
DISTAL TUBULE - Aldosterone stimulates; reabsorbs Na^+, kicks out K^+ or H^+.
COLLECTING TUBULE- with ADH = concentrated urine; without ADH = dilute urine, ↑ free H_2O excreted.

RENAL FAILURE
ACUTE RENAL FAILURE -Abrupt loss of renal function as demonstrated by ↑ BUN, ↑Creatinine, ↓ Urine
   output (Oliguria < 20 cc/hr, Anuria < 50 cc/24 hr), Dirty Urine Sediment.
• **PRERENAL**: DDX: Dehydration, blood loss, CHF, cardiogenic or septic shock, renal artery stenosis, burns,
   third spacing, nephrotic syndrome, cirrhosis, hepatorenal syndrome, dissecting aortic aneurysm, diuretics. DX:
   FE_{Na}^+ < 1; RFI <1; BUN/CR >20; U_{Na}^+ <10 mmol/L; U_{OSM} >500 mmol/kg H2O.
• **RENAL**: 75% of ARF is 2h to ATN. Better prognosis with toxic etiology than ischemic. DDX: ATN TRIAD:
   dehydration, infection, aminoglycoside. Others: nephrotoxins, malignant HTN, glomerulonephritis, SLE,
   vasculitis, post partum, interstitial nephritis, papillary necrosis, trauma, hemolytic uremic syndrome,
   scleroderma, rhabdomyolysis, preeclampsia .DX: Patchy necrosis, renal tubular casts, interstitial edema, ↑
   renin, hyperkalemia, metabolic acidosis, hyperphosphatemia, hypocalcemia, anemia. ESR, ANA, serum
   complement,antistreptolysin-Otiter.FE_{Na}^+ >1; RFI>1;BUN/CR <10-15;U_{Na}^+ >20mmol/L; U_{OSM} <250mmol/kg H_2O
• POST RENAL: Most commonly bladder neck, ureteral or urethral obstruction. DDX: Benign prostate
   hypertrophy, tumor, infection, nephro- or cystolithiasis, anticholinergics. DX: Sonography, IVP, retrograde
   pyelography. TREATMENT: Treat etiology and complications. Close monitoring and correction of abnormal
   electrolytes. Hyperkalemia is commonly seen. Keep K^+ <5.0 meq/L. Careful fluid therapy (ie UO + 400 ml/d), if
   hyponatremic may require more restrictions. Bicarbonate replacement may be necessary. Phosphate binders
   (Al hydroxide) prn. Low K^+ diet (<40 meq/D) or TPN. Continuous Arteriovenous hemofiltration, Hemo- or
   peritoneal dialysis if conservative management fails. Indications for dialysis: Hyperkalemia, resistant to
   aggressive treatment; Symptomatic volume overload, resistant to aggressive diuresis; Pericarditis; Uremic
   encephalopathy; Uncontrolled bleeding; Relative indication- creatinine >10 mg/dl and BUN > 100 mg/dl.

END STAGE RENAL DISEASE: The need for dialysis is based on a combination of factors: uremic symptoms
(usually BUN >100 mg/dl), creatinine >10mg/dl, Creatinine clearance 4-8 ml/min, hyperkalemia unresponsive
to medical treatment. Types of dialysis: Hemodialysis & peritoneal dialysis (CAPD, CCPD). Diet: protein
(CAPD 1-1.2 g/kg/d, Hemodialysis 0.8-1.0 g/kg/d), ↓ K, ↓ phosphorus. Other therapy -Iron (ferrous salts or IV
iron dextran) & folate supplements, phosphate binders, erythropoietin.

CHRONIC RENAL FAILURE: Differential Diagnosis: Nephrosclerosis, Diabetes mellitus, Primary
Glomerulopathy, NSAID/ Drug induced nephropathy, malignant HTN, Renal artery stenosis, Heavy metals.
Diagnosis: UA, Azotemia,↑ creatinine, sonography, IVP, renal Biopsy.

DIABETIC NEPHROPATHY

Stage	Renal Size	GFR (ml/min)	Albumin excretion	Arterial BP
I	Hypertrophy >14cm	≥150	<30mg/24h	Normal
II	Hypertrophy	150- 200	<30mg/24h	Normal
III	Normal, ≈ 12cm	130-150	30-300mg/24h	↑
IV	Reduced, ≤ 10cm	≤ 120	>300mg/24h	↑↑
V	Atrophic, <8cm	≤ 20	>3.5gm/24h	↑↑

NEPHROTIC SYNDROME
Edema; Hypercholesterolemia; Proteinuria >3.5 gm/24 hrs; hypertriglyceridemia; anasarca; hypoalbuminemia;
Lipiduria (oval fat bodies)
DDX: (* most common causes) *Primary glomerular disease , infections (ie *endocarditis, *HIV, mono, HBV),
drugs (gold, penicillamine, captopril, heroin, NSAIDS, *probenecid, mercury), neoplasia, misc. (SLE, *Henoch-
Schönlein purpura, *vasculitis, *sarcoidosis, amyloidosis, * Alport's syndrome, diabetes, *bee stings). DX:
Renal Biopsy, Serology Streptozyme, ANA, Complement, VDRL, Hep B AG; Heavy metals.

SIADH

Reabsorbs only free H_2O, not Na^+ = no edema. Draws water out of cells into extracellular fluid. Hyponatremia; Natriuresis; Hypouricemia; Volume expansion without edema; U_{osm} >300; U_{Na^+} >20-40meq; FE_{Na^+} >1; Normal BUN and Creatinine; ↓ serum osmolality

DDX: CNS disorders (traumatic, infectious), tumors (small cell lung, pancreas, Hodgkin's), pulmonary disorders (COPD, TB, infectious), endocrine disorders. Drugs (narcotics, NSAIDs vincristine, vinblastine, phenothiazine, tricyclics), hypothyroidism, positive pressure ventilation. TX: fluid restriction 800-1000 ml/d, (5% NaCl 300ml IV over 3-4h if severely confused, convulsions or coma)

CASTS

RBC: Yellow-orange, always significant. DDX: Toxic renal damage, Ischemic renal damage, Periarteritis Nodosa, Trauma, Embolism (Thromboembolism), Acute Glomerulonephritis.

HYALINE: Soft, clear cylinders. Not significant unless great numbers or with other casts.

WBC: Acute pyelonephritis, Lupus Nephritis, Interstitial Nephritis, Nephrotic Syndrome.

RENAL TUBULAR CAST: Damage to renal tubules. ATN, Chronic GN, Degenerative Vascular Disease.

FATTY: characteristic of nephrotic syndrome.

GRANULAR: fine or coarse, broken down renal tubular of WBC casts.

WAXY: colorless, sharp corners, frequently Broad (Chronic renal disease).

CRYSTALS: Calcium Oxalate, Calcium Oxalate/Phosphate, Mg, Ammonia Phosphate/Struvite.

DIURETIC EFFECTS

LOOP: most potent. Blocks Cl^- pump in ascending limb increasing Na^+/Cl in urine. Aldosterone tries to reclaim Na^+, kicks out K^+, eventually run out, kicks out H^+ resulting in Metabolic Alkalosis (Hypokalemic).

SPIRONOLACTONE: aldosterone antagonist, can cause increased K+.

THIAZIDES: works on distal tubule, inhibits Na^+/Cl reabsorption = Hypokalemic Metabolic Alkalosis (as above).

HEMATURIA

DDX: Coagulopathies, thrombocytopenia, UTI, kidney or bladder trauma, carcinoma, nephrolithiasis, prostatitis, urethritis, glomerulonephritis.

MISCELLANEOUS MEDICATIONS

basiliximab [Simulect] IV BID IL-2 receptor antagonist for organ rejection in renal transplant

daclizumab [Zenapax] IV 1 mg/kg IgG1 monoclonal antibody antagonist for organ rejection in renal transplant

Nephrology Notes:

NEUROLOGY EXAM

HISTORY - Rapid vs. Insidious onset; History of previous level of functioning from family and friends.

MENTAL STATUS SCREEN - Orientation (name, place, date); Observe speech (spontaneity & comprehension); Immediate recall (repeat 7 digit series); Recent memory (recall of 3 objects after 5 min.); Remote memory (recollection of history of illness); Reasoning abilities (serial 3's or 7's); REMEMBER: The majority of people are left sided brain dominant hemisphere = speech & math; Non-dominant hemisphere = sound localization, spatial orientation, body self-image.

CRANIAL NERVES

- **OLFACTORY (CN I)** - Tests: each nostril separately with familiar smells, avoiding noxious stimuli.
- **OPTIC (CN II)** - Tests: pupils to light (direct & consensual) & accommodation; test vision & visual fields.
- **OCULOMOTOR (CN III)** - Tests: Medial rectus adducts; Inferior rectus causes downward gaze; Superior rectus & Inferior oblique cause upward gaze.
- **TROCHLEAR (CN IV)** –Tests: Superior oblique causes the eye to internally rotate with downward and inward gaze
- **TRIGEMINAL (CN V)** – Tests: Direct corneal blink reflex; Cotton wisp for facial sensation; Tongue blade for oral mucosa and tongue sensation; Open & close jaw with & without resistance, palpate masseters.
- **ABDUCENS (VI)** – Tests: Lateral rectus abducts (lateral gaze).
- **FACIAL (CN VII)** Tests: Keep eyes closed against resistance; Smile; Consensual corneal blink reflex; Taste on anterior 2/3's of tongue; Sensory-skin of ear canal & behind ear; autonomic-submaxillary & sublingual salivary glands
- **ACOUSTIC (CN VIII)** – Tests: Finger rub & whisper for hearing; spontaneous nystagmus (eye moves slowly away from position of fixation, then corrected by a quick movement back-named first for fast component); Vertigo?
- **GLOSSOPHARYNGEAL (CN IX) & VAGUS (CN X)** – Tests: Assess elevation of uvula; Gag reflex; Assess swallow (if larynx rises) & voice for hoarseness.
- **ACCESSORY (CN XI)**- Tests: Rotation of head strength & shoulder shrug-palpate muscles during contraction
- **HYPOGLOSSAL (CN XII)** – Tests: Protrude tongue (deviates towards weak side).

MOTOR RESPONSE - General muscle strength, tone, & symmetry.

1. Heel drag: Pt. supine, quickly lift knee; normal heel will drag; suspect ↑'d muscle tone if heel lifts from table
2. Drift: Have Pt. extend arms directly in front, palms up, & close eyes; weakness results in one arm slowly drooping (sensitive indicator for minimally cooperative Pt.).
3. Screen muscle strength: Flex & extend wrist, forearm, & knee; plantar & dorsi flex ankle & great toe. Screen other muscle groups as indicated.
4. Grade muscle strength (Oxford scale):

Grade 0	No movement
Grade 1	Trace or flicker of contraction without joint movement
Grade 2	Partially moves about joint in absence of gravity
Grade 3	Moves against gravity, but, not applied pressure
Grade 4	Moves against gravity & some resistance
Grade 5	Full strength

5. Tremor - Oscillating movement about a joint due to involuntary contracting muscles, (all tremors disappear during sleep); resting or intentional?
6. Cogwheel rigidity - Jerking muscular resistance during passive movement of limb.
7. Choreiform movements - Rapid, purposeless, jerking movements.
8. Athetoid movements - Slower, writhing, asynchronous movements.
9. Hemiballismus - Sustained, violent, involuntary movements of limbs of one side of body.
10. Myoclonus - Single, or successive sudden jerks which may throw Pt. to floor.
11. Myotonia - continued contraction after voluntary or reflex act has ceased.

Respiratory Patterns

1. Kussmaul - deep regular breathing (metabolic acidosis),
2. Cheyne-Stokes - alternating periods of apnea & hyperpnea (regular, waxing & waning quality),
3. Biot - periods of apnea punctuated by a few deep breaths (irregular)

Sensory Exam - Least reliable.

1. Have Pt. outline area of sensory loss; if it is in a nerve root pattern - further testing may confirm Dx.
2. Test with cotton wisp lightly on skin (compare bilaterally & ask for discrepancy).
3. Hot/cold & vibration to extremities:compare lower with upper. Metabolic neuropathies tend to involve lower 1st
4. "Stocking/glove" paresis - consider a peripheral neuropathy.
5. "Cape like" paresis(across both upper extremities & upper chest) - consider lesion in spinal cord (syringomyelia, traumatic central cord syndrome, etc.).
6. Mixed sensory & opposite motor loss indicates partial spinal cord lesion (Brown-Sequard).

COORDINATION

1. Finger-nose: Pt. touches finger tip to examiner's finger to tip of nose in rapid succession. Tremor just before target is abnormal (cerebellar disease); wide oscillations or always precisely off target suggests hysteria.
2. Heel-shin: Pt. moves heel up & down shin. (Tests cerebellar & posterior column disease).
3. Alternating supinate-pronate of hands: Tests cerebellar disease. (Diadochokinesia: ability to arrest a motor impulse & substitute another).
4. Position of feet: Broad based stance may indicate spinocerebellar disease.
5. Cerebellar ataxia - Pt. stands with feet together & eyes open, (fall with cerebellar disease).
6. Romberg sign - stands with feet together & eyes closed; Tests for posterior column disease (proprioception).

Dermatomes

REFLEXES

DEEP TENDON REFLEXES: (2+ on scale of 4, or equal are considered normal)
• Biceps (C5-C6) *Musculocutaneous nerve*
• Brachioradialis (C5-C6) *Radial nerve*
• Triceps (C7-C8) *Radial nerve*
• Quadriceps (L2-L4) *Femoral nerve*
• Adductor (L2-L4) *Obturator nerve*
• Achilles (L5-S2) *Tibial nerve*

REFLEXES IN PYRAMIDAL TRACT DISEASE
• Muscle Clonus (ankle, patellar, & wrist)   • Hoffman's sign (flex distal phalanx index finger)
• Babinski's (dorsiflexed great toe, toes fan, dorsiflexed ankle, & flexion of knee & hip)
PRIMITIVE REFLEXES
• Grasp (cannot release grasp)   • Snout reflex (tap upper lip results in puckering/sucking)

COMA- Important Physical Findings

1. Color: cyanotic, pallor, icteric, cherry-red (CO poisoning)?
2. Head: contusions, depressions, battle's sign (ecchymoses behind ear), blood or CSF draining from ears or nose?
3. Eyes: pupils reactive & size (dilated or pinpoint), papilledema?
4. Facial muscles: one-sided droop?
5. Oral cavity: tongue lacerations (seizures), ulceration or discoloration from poisons?
6. Breath: alcohol, acetone, ammonia, other odors?
7. Neck: nuchal rigidity, Kernig's sign (flex hip & knee), Brudzinski's sign (flex neck)?
8. Posturing: <u>Decerebrate rigidity</u>: jaw clenched, neck retracted, arms & legs stiffly extended & internally rotated (brainstem involvement); <u>Decorticate rigidity</u>: arm(s) in flexion & adduction, leg(s) extended (lesions in cerebral white matter, internal capsules, & thalamus); <u>Diagonal posturing</u>: opposite arms & legs extended & flexed (?supratentorial lesions) OR extended arms and flexed legs (fragments of decerebrate posturing); <u>Abolition of all postures & movements</u>: acute bilateral corticospinal interruption & low pontine-medullary lesions.

GLASGOW COMA SCALE (GCS) (Prognostic indicator)- See EMERGENCY MEDICINE SECTION

CEREBROVASCULAR DISEASE

STROKE- Sudden, nonconvulsive, focal neurological deficit.
- Approximately 500,000 Americans a year suffer a new or recurrent stroke.
- Stroke is the 3rd leading cause of death in the United States.
- 25% of patients with a stroke die

RISK FACTORS:

MODIFIABLE: Hypertension, Diabetes, smoking, heart disease (coronary heart disease and heart failure doubles risk of stroke; atrial fibrillation, left sided chamber enlargement or aneurysm, transmural myocardial infarction, atrial myxoma, septic embolic, mitral valve disease), hyperlipidemia, hypercoagulable states (cancer, protein C & S deficiency, pregnancy), TIA (5% of patients with a TIA will have a completed stroke within a month if not treated with antiplatelet therapy), Polycythemia, Sickle cell anemia.

UNMODIFIABLE: Age (incidence increases in both men and women > 55 year of age), Gender (risk greater in men, although more women live to be >65 years and therefore more women than men over 65 die of stroke each year), Previous stroke (reoccurrence highest within 30 days of prior stroke; 4-14% per year thereafter), Heredity, Race (African Americans are twice as likely to die or be disabled from a stroke than Caucasians due to presence of more risk factors- sickle cell, smoking, hypertension, diabetes, hyperlipidemia)

CLASSIFICATION

ISCHEMIC: Account for ≈ 75% of strokes. Results from complete occlusion of an artery supplying an area of the brain due to Cerebral thrombosis (developing within the culprit artery) or embolism (forming elsewhere and then migrating to the brain). Anterior circulation (or carotid territory strokes) usually affect the cerebral hemispheres. Posterior circulation strokes (or vertebrobasilar territory strokes) usually affect the cerebellum or brainstem.

TIA (Transient Ischemic Attack) – Reversible episode of focal dysfunction of the brain or eye that is secondary to transient occlusion of an artery. 5% of patients with a TIA will have a completed stroke within a month if not recognized and treated. Symptoms are usually fleeting, lasting <10-15 minutes, 88% resolve within 1 hour. Initial attack most commonly presents with visual disturbances. Ipsilateral Amaurosis fugax (temporary, partial or complete monocular blindness) is a classic symptom of carotid artery TIA. Sensorimotor symptoms are contralateral. Rarely are the eye and brain involved simultaneously.

HEMORRHAGIC: Due to an arterial rupture resulting in an Intracerebral (bleeding into the parenchyma of the brain) or Subarachnoid bleed (bleeding onto the surface of the brain). Most common causes: Intracranial-hypertension, amyloid angiopathy; Subarachnoid- aneurysm >90%, AVM- 5%. Generally appear more ill and deteriorate more rapidly than those with ischemic stroke.

Subarachnoid: Sudden severe headache, "worst headache", generalized, may radiate to neck and face, may experience transient loss of consciousness. May have nausea, vomiting, photophobia, phonophobia, altered mental status.

Intracerebral: Sudden onset of focal neurological symptoms like patient with ischemic strokes, although are more likely to have decrease level of consciousness, headache and nausea and vomiting

Numbness and sensory deficits: Paresthesias occurs on the opposite side of the cerebral circulation involved. May cause tingling, sensory loss or other abnormal sensation in the face, arm, hand, or leg. May cause hemiparesthesia or all limbs may be affected.

Dysarthria: Abnormal pronunciation, slurring, mumbling and articulation of words.

Ataxia: Incoordination of one side of the body, poor balance, staggering gait.

Visual disturbances: Blurred vision in the left or right or both visual fields in both eyes. Diplopia- seeing two images. May have the sense of bouncing visual images. Ocular palsy- unable to move eyes to one side. Dysconjugate gaze- unable to move eye synchronously.

STROKE SYNDROMES

ANTERIOR CEREBRAL ARTERY (cerebral hemisphere, medial aspect)	
Signs and symptoms	Structures involved
Dyspraxia & tactile aphasia of left limbs	Corpus callosum
Gait apraxia	Frontal cortex
Paralysis of foot and leg with or without paresis of arm	Leg area with or without arm area of contralateral motor cortex
Sensory loss over toes, foot & leg	Foot and leg area of contralateral sensory cortex
Sucking and grasp reflexes	Medial surface of posterior frontal lobe
Urinary incontinence	Bilateral posteromedial aspect of superior frontal gyrus

MIDDLE CEREBRAL ARTERY (cerebral hemisphere, lateral aspect)	
Signs and symptoms	Structures involved
Agnosia for the left half of extra-personal space, constructional apraxia, dressing apraxia, impaired ability to judge distance, unilateral neglect, upside-down reading, visual illusions	parietal lobe- usually nondominant
Ataxia of limbs	Contralateral parietal lobe
Broca's aphasia (motor) (preserved comprehension; hesitant speech with word finding difficulty)	Motor speech area, dominant (usually left) frontal lobe
Conjugate gaze paralysis	Contralateral frontal contraversive field
Gaze preference, eyes deviated to side of the lesion	Frontal lobe, center for lateral gaze
Hemiparesis of face, arm more than leg	Contralateral parietal and frontal motor cortex-somatic motor area for face, arm and leg
Hemisensory deficit of face, arm & leg (cotton touch, pinprick, position, two point discrimination, vibration)	Contralateral somatosensory cortex area for face and arm and thalamoparietal projections
Homonymous hemianopia	Optic radiation
Pure motor hemiplegia	Int. capsule (upper, posterior limb)& corona radiata
Wernicke's aphasia (central), alexia, anomia, poor comprehension, jargon speech, word deafness Gerstmann syndrome (agraphia, acalculia, finger agnosia, right-left confusion)	Central speech area and parietoccipital cortex of dominant hemisphere

POSTERIOR CEREBRAL ARTERY	
Signs and symptoms	Structures involved
CEREBRAL HEMISPHERE, INFERIOR ASPECT:	
Bilateral hemianopsia, apraxia of ocular movements, cortical blindness, inability to count objects, inability to see movements to-and-fro, inability to perceive peripherally located objects, unaware of blindness	Bilateral occipital lobes
Cortical blindness	Occipital lobes, bilaterally
Dyslexia without agraphia, color anomia	Dominant calcarine cortex and posterior aspect of corpus callosum
Homonymous hemianopsia	Calcarine occipital cortex or optic radiation
Memory deficit	Hippocampus, dominant or bilaterally
Thalamic syndrome- Choreoathetosis, dense sensory loss, spontaneous pain & dysesthesias, spasms of hand, mild hemiparesis, intentional tremor	Thalamus (ventral posterolateral nucleus) & adjacent subthalamic nucleus
BRAINSTEM, MIDBRAIN:	
Contralateral hemiplegia	Cerebral peduncle
Convergence nystagmus, disorientation	Top of midbrain, periaqueductal
Decerebrate attacks	Motor tracts between red and vestibular nuclei
3rd nerve palsy and contralateral hemiplegia	3rd cranial nerve & cerebral peduncle (Weber's syn)
Paralysis/paresis of vertical eye movement	Supranuclear fibers to 3rd nerve
Thalamoperforate syndrome- superior, crossed cerebellar ataxia; Claude syndrome (inferior, crossed cerebellar ataxia with ipsilateral 3rd nerve palsy)	Dentatothalamic tract and 3rd nerve

VERTEBRAL ARTERY (brainstem, lateral medulla)	
Signs and symptoms	Structures involved
Ataxia, falling toward side of lesion	Cerebellar hemisphere or fibers
Dysphagia, hoarseness, vocal cord paralysis, decreased gag reflex	9th & 10th nerve
Horner's syndrome	Ipsilateral, descending sympathetic fibers
Numbness of arm and trunk	Ipsilateral cuneate and gracile nuclei
Pain and thermal sense impaired over half of body with or without face	Contralateral Spinothalamic tract
Vertigo, diplopia, nystagmus, nausea and vomiting	Vestibular nucleus

PONTOMEDULLARY BASILAR ARTERY (brainstem)	
Signs and symptoms	Structures involved
Abduction of eye paresis	Ipsilateral 6th nerve
Ataxia	Middle cerebellar peduncle and cerebellum
Blindness, impaired acuity, visual field defects	Visual cortex
Coma	Tegmentum of midbrain, thalami
Conjugate gaze paresis	Ipsilateral center for lateral gaze
Diplopia, internuclear ophthalmoplegia, horizontal &/or vertical nystagmus, conjugate lateral &/or vertical gaze paralysis	Ocular motor nerves, medial longitudinal fasciculus, vestibular and conjugate gaze apparatus
Facial paralysis	Ipsilateral 7th nerve
Hemifacial sensory deficit	Ipsilateral descending tract and nucleus of V
Horner's syndrome (miosis, ptosis, decreased sweating)	Descending sympathetic pathways
Pain and thermal sense diminished over half of body with or without face	Contralateral Spinothalamic tract
Paralysis or weakness of all extremities & all bulbar muscles	Corticospinal and corticobulbar tracts bilaterally

PEARLS

AMAUROSIS FUGAX- transient monocular blindness most commonly due to stenosis of the ipsilateral carotid artery. May also be caused by embolism of retinal arteries or idiopathic.

APHASIA	Fluent	Comprehension	Repetition
Broca's	no	good	poor
Transcortical motor	no	good	good
Global	no	poor	poor
Mixed transcortical	no	poor	good
Wernicke	yes	poor	poor
Transcortical sensory	yes	poor	good
Conduction	yes	good	poor
Anomic	yes	good	good

CARPAL TUNNEL SYNDROME- Compression of the median nerve at the wrist. Most commonly due to excessive use of the hand or repeated occupational trauma. Paresthesias tend to be worse at night. Impaired superficial sensory to the thumb, 2nd, 3rd and may involve 1/2 of the 4th finger. Pain may radiate to the elbow and shoulder. Atrophy of the abductor pollicis brevis is a late finding. Electrophysiologic testing is diagnostic.

GUILLAIN-BARRE' SYNDROME (Acute Inflammatory Polyneuropathy, Acute Autoimmune Neuropathy) Cause unknown (thought to be a cell mediated reaction against the peripheral nerve). Common form of polyneuropathy, most rapidly developing and fatal form. All ages, female >male, all seasons. Symmetrical weakness develops over days to weeks, lower extremity usually first. Myalgia, paresthesias, hypotonia, reduced or absent reflexes, autonomic dysfunction, respiratory failure. DX: CSF- acellular, high protein, normal pressure; EMG- reduced conduction velocity, prolonged distal latencies. TX: Ventilatory assistance, plasmapheresis; immune globulin

HEADACHE- Migraine: throbbing, pulsatile unilateral or bilateral frontotemporal, 4-24h; provoking factors- light, noise, tension, alcohol; Associated symptoms- nausea, vomiting, scotomas, blindness, scintillating lights, unilateral numbness, weakness, vertigo, confusion, dysphasia. Cluster: intense orbital-temporal non-throbbing, occurring nightly more than daily for weeks and may reoccur after months or years; Associated symptoms- rhinorrhea, lacrimation, conjunctival injection. Tension: pressure, tight aching generalized headache; Provoking factors- anxiety, fatigue.

HUNTINGTON'S CHOREA- Triad of dominant inheritance, dementia and choreoathetosis. Impaired glucose metabolism in the caudate nucleus and atrophy. Abnormal movements thought to be due to a heightened sensitivity of striatal dopamine receptors and dopamine excess.

LAMBERT-EATON SYNDROME- Decreased presynaptic release of acetylcholine. Fatigue improves with exercise. Associated with malignancy in 60% of the cases (most commonly small cell lung cancer).

MENINGITIS- Common presentation nuchal rigidity, leukocytosis, fever, headache, coma. Start empiric antimicrobials if the diagnosis is considered (DON'T wait until work up is complete). DX: Lumbar puncture (perform CT first if focal neurological deficit is found), CT of head (if unsure of history or physical findings to rule out structural pathology), blood cultures. Distinguish between bacterial, viral and fungal. Most common bacterial causes by age group: Neonate- group B or D streptococci, Enterobacteriaceae; Infant 1-3mo- H. influenzae, Pneumococci, Meningococci, group B or D streptococci; Child 3mo-7yr- H. influenzae, Pneumococci, Meningococci, Adult (>7yr)- Pneumococci, Meningococcal, Listeria monocytogenes.

PUPILS- pupilloconstrictor- fibers arise in Edinger-Westphal nucleus in the midbrain then travel through the 3rd nerve to the ciliary ganglion in the orbit. Pupillodilator- posterolateral hypothalamus to 8th cervical and 1st & 2nd thoracic segments to lateral horn cells to the 1st division of trigeminal nerve to long ciliary nerve. Adie pupil: blurred vision and myosis, decreased reaction to light, better response to near due to degeneration of the ciliary ganglion and post ganglionic parasympathetic fibers. Argyll Robertson pupil: fail to react to light, constricts on accomodation, usually due to syphilis. Marcus Gunn pupil: absent or slowed direct pupil constriction to bright light with pupillary escape (failure to sustain pupillary constriction) due to ipsilateral optic nerve disease. Consensual constriction to the involved eye remains intact with bright light stimulation to the uninvolved eye.

INTERNATIONAL CLASSIFICATION OF EPILEPTIC SEIZURES
I. Partial seizures (focal, local)
A. Simple Partial Seizures (unimpaired consciousness)
    1. with motor symptoms
    2. with somatosensory or special sensory symptoms
    3. with autonomic symptoms
    4. with psychic symptoms

B. Complex partial seizures (with impaired consciousness)
    1. Beginning as simple partial seizures & progressing to impaired consciousness
      a. without other features
      b. with features in I.A.1 to I.A.4
      c. with automatisms
    2. With impairment of consciousness at onset
      a. without other features
      b. with features in I.A.1 to I.A.4
      c. with automatisms
C. Partial seizures evolving to secondarily generalized seizures
    1. Simple partial seizures evolving to generalized seizures
    2. Complex partial seizures evolving to generalized seizures
    3. Simple partial seizures evolving to complex partial seizures to generalized seizures
II. Generalized seizures (convulsive or nonconvulsive)
A. Absence seizures
    1. Absence seizures
    2. Atypical absence seizures
B. Myoclonic seizures
C. Clonic seizures
D. Tonic seizures
E. Tonic-clonic seizures
F. Atonic seizures (astatic seizures)
III. Unclassified epileptic seizures

ALZHEIMER'S DISEASE
donepezil HCl [Aricept] (Tab 5,10 mg) Alzheimer's Disease PO 5 mg QD before bed for 4-6wks then may increase to 10 mg qhs if needed
Hydergine [ergoloid mesylates] (sublingual Tab 0.5 mg) initial dose is 1 mg TID. Doses up to 4.5 to 12 mg/day, Up to 6 months of treatment may be necessary to determine efficacy, using doses of at least 6 mg/day.
tacrine HCl [Cognex] (Tab 10, 20, 30, 40 mg) Alzheimer's Disease PO 10 mg QID for first 6wks, must monitor serum transaminase level weekly for 18 weeks then q 3 months & weekly for 6 weeks after dosing changes

ANESTHETICS

bupivacaine [Marcaine, Sensorcaine] *Local* 0.25%; *Peripheral nerve blocks* 0.5%, 0.25%; *Dental* 0.5% with epi.

chloroprocaine [Nesacaine] 1%, 2%; without preservatives 2%, 3%

EMLA [lidocaine 2.5% and prilocaine 2.5%] (Cream 5, 30 gm tubes; disc 2.5 inch) apply a thick layer of cream to intact skin and cover with an occlusive dressing, or an EMLA anesthetic disc is applied to intact skin. <u>Adult:</u> For minor procedures (ie. IV cannulation, venipuncture) apply 2.5 grams over 20-25 cm ^{2} of skin surface, or 1 Anesthetic Disc (1g over 10 cm ^{2}) for > 1 h. For more painful procedures involving a larger skin area (ie. split thickness skin graft harvesting) apply 2 grams of cream per 10 cm ^{2} of skin for at least 2 hours. Adult male genital skin: as an adjunct prior to local anesthetic infiltration, apply a thick layer of cream (1g/10cm ^{2}) to the skin surface for 15 minutes. Administer local anesthetic infiltration immediately after removal of cream.
<u>Pediatric:</u>**MAX** dose, area and application time:0-3 months or <5 kg: 1 g, 10 cm ^{2}, 1 h; 3-12 months and >5 kg: 2 g, 20 cm ^{2}, 4 h; 1-6 yr and >10 kg: 10 g, 100 cm ^{2}, 4 h; 7 to 12 yr and >20 kg: 20 g, 200 cm ^{2}, 4 h ★

etidocaine [Duranest] (20 & 30cc vials of 1.0 & 1.5% solutions)

lidocaine [Xylocaine] *Nerve block* 0.5%, 1%, 1.5%, 2% with or without epi; *Maximum doses of Xylocaine:* without epinephrine 4.5 mg/kg, with epi 7 mg/kg; 1% Xylocaine is 10 mg/ml, 2% Xylocaine is 20 mg/ml (Amide class)

mepivacaine [Carbocaine] *Local* 0.5%, 1%; *Peripheral nerve blocks* 1%, 2%; (Amide)

procaine [Novocaine] *Local* 1.0% *Maximum doses:* without epinephrine 7 mg/kg, with epi 9 mg/kg; *Spinal Anesthesia* 10% (Ester class)

ropivacaine [Naropin] (Inj 2, 5, 7.5, 10 mg/ml) Varies with procedure

GENERAL ANESTHETICS

ketamine HCl [Ketalar] (10, 50, 100 mg/ml inj) 1-4.5 mg/kg SIVP (duration 5-10mins); 6.5-13mg/kg IM (duration 12-25mins.); *Maintenance:* use 1/2-1 times the induction dose as needed.

methohexital sodium [Brevital] (0.5, 2.5, 5g inj) *Induction:* 50-120 mg SIVP(1ml/5secs)with duration 5-7mins. *Maintenance:* 20-40 mg SIVP q 4-7mins, OR, 3ml of a 0.2% solution/min continuous IV drip, titrate to effect.

propofol [Diprivan] (10 mg/ml in 20 & 50ml vials) 0.3-200 mcg/kg/min; *ICU sedation:* the average infusion rate was 27 mcg/kg/min for all Pts. (Age & concomitant use of other sedatives generally require less).

thiopental sodium [Pentothal] (20, 25 mg/ml inj; 400 mg/g rectal susp) *Anesthesia:* 50-75 mg IVP over 20-40secs, followed by 25-50 mg SIVP whenever the Pt moves. *Convulsive states:* 75-250 mg SIVP.

ANALEPTICS

doxapram [Dopram] (20 mg/ml injectable) 0.5-1mg/kg as single IV injection.

AMPHETAMINES C-II

amphetamine sulfate (5, 10 mg tablets) *Narcolepsy* use 5-60 mg/day in divided doses; ADD use 2.5-5 mg QD-BID; Exogenous obesity use 5-30 mg daily in divided doses.

dextroamphetamine sulfate [Dexedrine] dose as amphetamine sulfate above.

methamphetamine HCl [Desoxyn] (5 mg tablet; 5, 10, 15 mg long-acting tablet) *ADD* use 5 mg QD-BID initially, then titrate up to optimum response (usually 20-25 mg daily); Obesity use 5 mg 30min before meals.

Biphetamine 12½, 20 [dextroamphetamine/amphetamine] (Capsules: 12½ - 6.25/6.25 mg; 20 - 10/10 mg) Once daily dosing, titrate with Dexedrine for optimum dose.

ANOREXIANTS

benzphetamine C3 [Didrex] (Tab 25, 50 mg) PO 25-50 mg mid-morning, increase to BID/TID if needed

dexfenfluramine [Redux] ★★ withdrawn from the market in SEP 97 pending further investigation

dextroamphetamine C2 [Dexedrine] (Tab 5, 10 mg) PO 5-10 mg TID 30-60min before meals

diethylpropion HCl C4 [Tenuate, Tepanil] (Tab 25 mg) PO 25 mg TID 1h before meal and in mid-evening

diethylpropion HCl [Tenuate Dospan] (Tab 75 mg) PO 75 mg once daily, in midmorning

fenfluramine C4 [Pondimin] ★★ withdrawn from the market in SEP 97 pending further investigation

mazindol C4 [Mazanor, Sanorex] (Tab 1,2 mg) PO 1 mg TID 1h before meals or 2 mg QD 1h before lunch

methamphetamine C2 [Desoxyn] (Tab 5 mg) PO 5 mg TID 30min before meals

phendimetrazine C3 [Plegine] (Tab 35 mg) PO 17.5-35 mg BID/TID 1h before meals

phendimetrazine HCl C2 [Preludin] (Tab 75 mg) PO 75 mg QD

phendimetrazine tartrate C3 [Prelu-2] (Tab/Cap 35 mg SR 105 mg) PO 35 mg BID-TID or SR 1 QD in AM

phentermine HCl C4 [Fastin] (Tab 8, 15, 18.75, 30, 37.5mg) PO 1 tab QD 1h before breakfast or 10h before HS

sibutramine C4 [Meridia](Cap 5, 10, 15 mg) Adults ≥16yoa use 10 mg QD; after 4 weeks may use 15 mg QD

ANTICONVULSANTS

<u>acetazolamide</u> (Tab 125, 250 mg; 500 mg/vial) 8-30 mg/kg/day

<u>carbamazepine</u> [Tegretol] (Chw 100 mg; Tab 200 mg; Susp 100 mg/5cc; XR 100, 200, 400 mg) ADULTS Begin with 200 mg BID or 1 tsp QID. Increase weekly up to 100 mg/d (using BID with XR or TID/QID with others) to best response to max of 1200 mg/d. PEDS (6-12yrs) Begin with 100 mg BID or ½ tsp QID & increase as above to max of 1000 mg/d. PEDS (<6yrs) Begin with 10-20 mg/kg/d as Tabs BID or TID or Susp QID; *increase* weekly TID/QID to max of 35 mg/kg/d

<u>clonazepam</u> [Klonopin] (Tab 0.5, 1, 2 mg) Initially 0.5 mg TID, increase 1mg every 3 days to a max of 20 mg/d

<u>clorazepate</u> [Tranxene] (Cap 3.75, 7.5,15 mg, Tab 3.75, 7.5,11.25,15, 22.5 mg) 7.5mg TID,↑ 7.5 mg/wk, max of 90 mg/d

<u>Carbatrol</u> [carbamazepine extended release] (Cap 200, 300 mg) PO see carbamazepine- same daily dose given BID

<u>Diastat</u> [diazepam] (rectal gel 2.5, 5, 10, 15, 20 mg/applicator) Age 2-5yrs 0.5 mg/kg/dose; 6-11yrs 0.3 mg/kg/dose; ≥12yrs 0.2 mg/kg/dose; May repeat dose in 4-12hrs

<u>diazepam</u> [Valium] (Tab 2, 5, 0 mg) PO 2-10 mg BID/TID/QID,IV 5-10 mg q10-15min up to 30 mg, may repeat in 2-4h

<u>ethosuximide</u> [Zarontin] (Cap 250 mg; Syp 250 mg/5cc) Initially use: (3-6 yrs) 250 mg/24h; (≥6 yrs) 500 mg/24h

<u>ethotoin</u> [Peganone] (Tab 250, 500 mg Initial dose ≤1g daily, titrate up to 2-3g daily

<u>felbamate</u> [Felbatol] (Tab 400, 600 mg; Susp 600 mg/5cc) 3600 mg/day. **FDA recommends use be suspended due to reported cases of aplastic anemia, unless, in the physician's judgment there is no other alternative therapy for a given patient and the benefits are greater than the risks of stopping felbamate, October 1994.

<u>fosphenytoin</u> [Cerebyx] (Vials 150{100 PE), 750{500 PE}mg) IV *status epilepticus* 15-20 mg phenytoin sodium equivalents (PE)/kg at rate of 100-150 PE/min, Non emergent IM/IV 10-20 mg PE/kg, maintenance 4-6 mg PE/kg/d

<u>gabapentin</u> [Neurontin] (Cap 100, 300, 400 mg) 900-1800 mg/day in 3 divided doses.

<u>lamotrigine</u> [Lamictal] (Tab 25, 100, 150, 200 mg) Adults >16yr: 50 mg/d for 2 wk, then 100 mg/d for 2 wk then 300-500 mg/d in 2 divided doses. In combination with valproate: 25 mg/d wks 1-4 then 100-150 mg/d

<u>magnesium sulfate</u> (12.5%=1mEq/ml, 50%=4mEq/ml) (1g=8.12mEq) 4-5g IM/IV q 4h; IV 1.5ml/min of 10% sol, OR, mix in 250cc D5 or NS & give 3ml/min.

<u>mephenytoin</u> [Mesantoin] (Tab 100 mg) 50-100 mg/24h first week, then titrate to 200-600 mg/24h.

<u>methsuximide</u> [Celontin] (Cap 150, 300 mg) Begin with 300 mg/day, advance at weekly intervals to a max of 1.2g/d

<u>paramethadione</u> [Paradione] (Cap 150, 300 mg) 900 mg-2.4g/d divided TID-QID.

<u>phenacemide</u> [Phenurone] (Tab 500 mg) Begin with 500 mg TID.

<u>phenobarbital</u> [Luminal] 60-100 mg/day PO; 200-320 mg IM/IV may repeat in 6h

<u>phensuximide</u> [Milontin] (Cap 500 mg) 500-1000 mg BID-TID

<u>phenytoin</u> [Dilantin] (Inj 50 mg/ml; Chw 50 mg; Susp 30, 125 mg/5cc; Cap 30, 100 mg; extended release 30, 100 mg) *Status epilepticus* use 10-15 mg/kg IV, do not exceed 50 mg/min. Loading dose use 1 g divided as 400 mg, 300 mg, 300 mg at 2h intervals, then 100 mg TID, OR, 300 mg extended tabs once daily

<u>primidone</u> [Mysoline] (Tab 50, 250 mg Susp 250 mg/5cc)100-125 mg gradually increased from QD to BID, TID/QID

<u>Tegretol-XR</u> [carbamazepine extended release] (Tab 100, 200, 400 mg) PO see carbamazepine- same daily dose given BID

<u>tiagabine</u> [Gabitril] (Tab 4, 12, 16, 20 mg) Initial dose for age 12-18 & adult use 4 mg QD, titrate dose at weekly intervals as follows: *Children 12-18 yoa* add 4 mg week 2, then may increase 4-8 mg QD at weekly intervals up to Max 32 mg/day. *Adults >18 yoa* add 4-8 mg QD at weekly intervals up to Max 56 mg/day.

<u>topiramate</u> [Topamax] (Tabs 25, 100, 200 mg) 400 mg/day in divided doses

<u>trimethadione</u> [Tridione] (Chw 150 mg; Cap 300 mg; Sol 40 mg/cc) 900 mg-2.4g/day divided TID-QID

<u>valproic acid</u> [Depakene (Cap 250 mg; Syp 250 mg/5cc) Depakote (Delayed rel tab 125, 250, 500 mg; Sprinkles 125 mg)] Initially, 15 mg/kg/d divided BID/TID with food; ↑weekly 5-10 mg/kg/d prn to max of 60 mg/kg/d [Deparon] (5ml vial): IV administer as a 60 min infusion (≤20 mg/min) same frequency as the oral.

MIGRAINE

<u>Cafergot</u> [ergotamine tartrate/caffeine] (Tab 1mg/100 mg; Supp 2 mg/100 mg) 2 tabs followed by 1 tab q ½ hr to a max of 6 tabs/attack; OR, a max of 2 supp/attack.

<u>dihydroergotamine mesylate</u> [DHE 45] (1mg/ml) IM/IV 1mg q1h to a max of 3mg IM & 2 mg IV. Unlabeled use: metoclopramide 10 mg + DHE 1mg IM MAX of 3 mg

<u>dihydroergotamine mesylate</u> [Migranal] (NS 0.5 mg/spray) 1 spray each nostril; repeat 15 mins later. Max 6 sprays/24 hrs and 8 sprays/week.

<u>ergotamine</u> [Ergostat, Medihaler] (Tab 2 mg sublingual, Inh 0.36mg/dose) 1 tab SL q 30 min X 3 doses/24h max.; inh 1 inhalation, may repeat in 5 minutes, MAX 6 inh/24h

<u>methysergide</u> [Sansert] (Tab 2 mg) 4-8 mg daily with meals. SE: Retroperitoneal fibrosis

<u>Midrin</u> [isometheptene/dichloralphenazone/acetaminophen, 65 mg/100 mg/325 mg capsule] 2 capsules followed by 1 capsule q 1h to a MAX of 5/12h. Tension HA 1-2 capsules q 4h, MAX 8/24h

<u>naratriptan</u> [Amerge] (Tab 1, 2.5 mg) PO 1-2.5 mg may repeat in 4h, Max 5 mg/24 h; serotonin 5-HT 1 receptor Agonists

<u>rizatriptan</u> [Maxalt, Maxalt-MLT] (Tab 5, 10 mg) PO 5-10 mg may repeat Q 2h, Max 30 mg/24 h

<u>sumatriptan</u> [Imitrex] (Tab 25, 50 mg; Inj 6mg/.5cc unit dose; NS 5 & 20 mg/unit dose spray devices) PO 1 Tab at onset, then may repeat in 2h, MAX 12/24h; SC, may repeat in 1h. Max 12 mg/24h. Nasal Spray (NS) use 5, 10, or 20 mg administered in one nostril, may repeat in 2 hours. (10 mg dose – give 5 mg in each nostril). Max 40 mg/day

<u>zolmitriptan</u> [Zomig] (Tabs 2.5, 5 mg) *Adults use* 2.5 mg or lower at start of migraine, may repeat in 2 hrs. Max 10 mg/day & 3 treatments in a 30 day period. 5-HT$_{1B/1D}$ receptor antagonist

NEUROMUSCULAR BLOCKERS

<u>atracurium besylate</u> [Tracrium] (10 mg/ml) *Tracheal Intubation* use 0.4-0.5 mg/kg IVP (avg onset: 2-2.5min; avg duration: 20-45min), follow with 0.08-0.1mg/kg IVP q 15-25min, OR, 2-15 mcg/kg/min cont IV infusion.

<u>cisatracurium</u> [Nimbex] (2mg/ml, 10 mg/ml) *Adults* 0.1mg/kg IV initial dose followed by 0.5-10.2 mcg/kg/min infusion (average rate 3 mcg/kg/min)★

<u>doxacurium chloride</u> [Nuromax] (1mg/ml) *Tracheal Intubation*: 0.05-0.08 mg/kg IVP (avg onset: 5min; avg duration:≈100-160min), follow with 0.005-0.01mg/kg IVP q ≈30-45min.

<u>gallamine triethiodide</u> [Flaxedil] (20 mg/ml) 1-1.5 mg/kg (MAX 100 mg) IV. Produces 50-75% ↓ in minute vol

<u>hexafluorenium bromide</u> [Mylaxen] (20 mg/ml) *Adjunctively prolongs succinylcholine neuromuscular blockade.* 0.4mg/kg IV, 3 mins later, follow with 0.2 mg/kg succinylcholine IV. (avg onset: 3-4min; avg duration: 20-30min).

<u>mivacurium</u> [Mivacron] (0.5 mg/ml, 2 mg/ml inj) *Tracheal Intubation* use 0.15 mg/kg IVP over 5-15 sec (avg onset: 2.5 min; avg duration: 25-30 min); maintenance dose - 0.1mg/kg IVP for extra 15 mins.

<u>pancuronium</u> [Pavulon] (1mg/ml, 2 mg/ml) *Adults & Children* use 0.04-0.1mg/kg IV, ↑ incrementally 0.01mg/kg for prolonged blockade. *Tracheal Intubation*: 0.06-0.1mg/kg IVP (avg onset: 2-3 min; avg duration: 22-65 min).

<u>pipecuronium bromide</u> [Arduan] (1mg/ml) *Tracheal Intubation*: 0.07-0.085 mg/kg IVP (avg onset: 2.5-3 min; avg duration: 1-2hrs),follow with 0.01-0.015mg/kg IVP q ≈50mins. *Base dosage on Ideal Body Weight if >30% IBW*

<u>rocuronium</u> [Zemuron] (10 mg/ml) *Tracheal Intubation*: 0.45-1.2 mg/kg IVP, (avg onset: 0.4-6 min; avg duration: 15-160min); maintenance dose-0.1-0.2 mg/kg IVP or Cont. IV infusion at 0.01-0.012 mg/kg/min based on TOF

<u>succinylcholine chloride</u> [Anectine, Quelicin, Sucostrin] (20, 50, 100 mg/ml) *Tracheal Intubation*: 1-2.5 mg/kg (MAX 150 mg) IVP (avg onset: 30-60sec; avg duration: 4-6min), *May use* 3-4mg/kg IM *for PEDS when vein inaccessible.* Continuous IV infusion at 0.5-10 mg/min.

<u>vecuronium bromide</u> [Norcuron] (1mg/ml, 2 mg/ml) *Tracheal Intubation*: 0.08-0.1mg/kg (MAX 0.28 mg/kg) IVP (avg onset: 2.5-3min; avg duration: 25-30min), follow with 0.010-0.015 mg/kg IVP q 12-15min, OR, 1 mcg/kg/min cont IV infusion.

PARKINSONIAN AGENTS

<u>amantadine</u> [Symmetrel] (Cap 100 mg; Syp 50 mg/5cc) 100 mg BID when used alone.

<u>benztropine mesylate</u> [Cogentin] (Tab 0.5, 1, 2 mg; Inj 1mg/ml) 1-6mg/day PO/IV.

<u>biperiden</u> [Akineton] (Tab 2 mg; Inj 5 mg/ml) 2 mg TID-QID up to 16mg/24h.

<u>bromocriptine</u> [Parlodel] (Tab 2.5 mg; Cap 5 mg) Initially1.25 mg BID with meals, increase 2.5 mg/day q 2-4 weeks to 10-40 mg/d

<u>carbidopa</u> [Lodosyn] (Tab 25 mg) titrate with levodopa

<u>diphenhydramine</u> [Benadryl] (Tab 25-50 mg 3-4 times daily

<u>ethopropazine</u> [Parsidol] (Tab 10, 50 mg) 50-600 mg QD

<u>levodopa</u> [Larodopa, Dopar] (Tab 100, 250, 500 mg; Cap 100, 250, 500 mg) 0.5-1 g daily in 2 divided doses, increase 0.75 g/d q 3-7 days to a max dose of 8 g/day

<u>pergolide</u> [Permax] (Tab 0.05, 0.25, 1mg) Initially, 0.05 mg QD X 2days, then increase 0.1-0.15 mg/day every 3rd day to a mean therapeutic dose of 3mg/day usually divided TID

<u>pramipexole</u> [Mirapex] (Tab 0.125, 0.25, 1, 1.5 mg) *Initially* 0.125 mg TID, ↑every 5-7 days. MAX 1.5 mg TID

<u>procyclidine</u> [Kemadrin] (Tab 5 mg) 2.5 mg TID PC, may increase to 5 mg TID PC

<u>ropinirole</u> [Requip] (Tab 0.25, 0.5, 1, 2, 5 mg) PO initial 0.25 mg three times daily, after 4 weeks may increase weekly by 1.5 mg/d up to a dose of 9 mg/day, then by <= 3 mg/d weekly to a total dose of 24 mg/d

<u>selegiline</u> [Carbex ;Eldepryl] (Tab 5 mg; Cap 5 mg) 5 mg with Breakfast & lunch daily.

<u>Sinemet</u> [carbidopa/levodopa] (Tab 10/100, 25/100, 25/250 mg; CR 25/100, 50/200 mg) 10/100 tid- qid, 25/100 tid; CR 25/100, 50/200 mg bid; titrate or change ratio as needed

<u>tolcapone</u> [Tasmar] (Tab 100, 200 mg) PO initial 100 mg TID; maintenance 100-200 mg TID, first dose of the day given with the levodopa/carbidopa dose; adjunct to levodopa/carbidopa therapy; ALT & AST baseline then Q2 weeks for 1st year then Q4 weeks for 6 mo then every 8 weeks

<u>trihexyphenidyl</u> [Artane] (Tab 2, 5 mg; SR Cap 5 mg; Elx 2 mg/ml) 1-2 mg day one, increase by 2 mg/3-5 days to total of 6-10 mg daily. Use SR for maintenance.

MISCELLANEOUS

Avonex [Interferon beta-1a] (33 mcg/vial) >18yoa use 30 mcg IM once weekly. *multiple sclerosis*

glatiramer acetate [Copaxone] (vial 20 mg) 20 mg SC daily. *multiple sclerosis*

Neurology Notes:

ASSESSING PROTEIN-ENERGY MALNUTRITION

	Moderate PEM	Severe PEM
% weight loss	15-25	>25
Fat depletion (triceps skin fold)	<16±6	<12±5
Serum albumin ($t^{1/2}$ 18-20 days)*	2.5-3.0	<2.5
Transferrin ($t^{1/2}$ 8-9 days)	1-2.0	<1
Prealbumin ($t^{1/2}$ 2-3 days)	5-9	<5
Total lymphocyte count	0.8-1.2	<0.8
Delayed hypersensitivity index	1	0

*Serum albumin - Normal (3.5-5.0 g/dl); Mild depletion (3.0-3.4). During periods of stress (surgery, burns, inf, trauma, etc.), albumin is used as an energy source. So, during these acute episodes, albumin does not indicate malnutrition.

METHODS FOR ESTIMATING CALORIC NEEDS

I. *Indirect Calorimetry* – uses monitor attached to respiratory quotient and energy expenditure based on O_2 consumption & CO_2 production.

II. *Harris-Benedict estimation of Basal Metabolic Rate (BMR) in kcal/day*

BMR (men) = 66 + (13.7 X W*) + (5 X H) - (6.8 X A)

BMR (women) = 655 + (9.7 X W*) + (1.8 X H) - (4.7 X A)

W = IBW(kg)*, H = height(cm), A = age(years)

Activity factors:
Hospitalized patients = 1.3
Non-hospitalized patients, active = 1.5

*Ideal Body Weight (IBW) female = 100lbs for 1st 5ft + 5lbs for every inch over 5 ft
male = 106lbs for 1st 5ft + 6lbs for every inch over 5 ft
(subtract 2lbs for each inch under 5 ft)
Adjusted IBW for obesity (Wt >125% IBW) = 0.25(Current BW - IBW) + IBW
Adjusted IBW for amputations = subtract following factors from IBW: 1.8% foot; 3.1% forearm; 0.8% hand; 7.1% BKA; 6.5% arm & shoulder; 13.4% AKA; 18.5% lower extremity.

Total Daily Caloric Needs = BMR(or adjusted BMR) X activity factor

III. *Weight Based Estimation*

Activity	kcal/lb	kcal/kg
Weight reduction	9-11.4	20-25
Bedrest (non-stressed)	11.4-13.6	25-30
Light (routine activities, mild stress)	13.6-16	30-35
Moderate (reg exercise, hypercatabolism)	16-20.5	35-45
Vigorous (heavy worker, athlete, trauma, burns)	20.5-22.7	45-50

METHODS FOR ESTIMATING PROTEIN NEED (1 g protein = 6.25 g N)

I. *Grams protein per kilogram*

RDA for normal healthy adult.................... 0.8-1.0 g/kg IBW
Mild to moderate stress .... 1.5 g/kg IBW
Severe stress... 2.0 g/kg IBW
Burns... ≥2.0 g/kg IBW
Renal failure (Chronic Renal Failure) .... 0.6-0.8 g/kg IBW
Renal Failure (hemodialysis) .... 1.1-1.4 g/kg IBW
Renal failure (CAPD) .... 1.2-1.5 g/kg IBW
Renal failure (CAVH) .... 1.5-1.8 g/kg IBW
Liver disease (no encephalopathy) .... 1.0-1.5 g/kg dry wt.
Liver disease (with encephalopathy)........ 40 g/day, ↑ 10-15 g/day to 0.8-1.0 g/kg as mental status improves
Liver disease (coma).................................. 0 g protein

II. *Nitrogen(N) Balance using UUN (24° Urinary Urea Nitrogen) (requires normal renal function for accuracy)*

$$\text{N balance} = \text{N input} - \text{N output} = \frac{\text{protein intake(g)}}{6.25} - (\text{UUN} + 4)$$

Negative N balance = catabolism; Zero N balance = maintenance; Positive N balance = anabolism

(UUN + 4) + desired N balance X 6.25 = g protein needed to achieve desired N balance

PARENTERAL NUTRITION

STEP 1: Determine total daily caloric needs, STEP 2. Determine protein needs, STEP 3. Calculate lipids based on 30-40% of total calories, STEP 4. Estimate fluid needs (typically 35 ml/kg/24° for avg. person – varies with clinical condition), STEP 5. Calculate amount of dextrose needed to complete total caloric needs, vary concentration to arrive at appropriate fluid need (ex: 700 kcal ≅ 206 g CHO≅500 cc of 41% dextrose≅750 cc of 27% dextrose)

Components: *amino acids* [various conc% & formulations] = volume X conc%/100 = g protein; 4 kcal/g protein
Dextrose [70%, can be diluted] conc%/100 X volume = g CHO; 3.4 kcal/g CHO;
Lipids [10, 20%] conc%/100 X volume = g lipids; 9 kcal/g lipid;
Electrolytes Na⁺Cl, Na⁺HCO₃, Na⁺lactate, Na⁺phosphate; K⁺acetate, KCl, K⁺phosphate; Ca²⁺Cl, Ca²⁺gluconate, Ca²⁺gluceptate; Mg²⁺sulfate, Mg²⁺Cl; Ammonium chloride.
Vitamins [1 amp MVI-12 = 10cc] vit C 100 mg; vit A 3300 IU; vit D 200 IU; thiamine 3 mg; riboflavin 3.6 mg; niacinamide 40 mg; pyridoxine 4 mg; dexpanthenol 15 mg; vit E 10 IU; biotin 60 µg; folic acid 400 µg; cyanocobalamin 5 g. May add extra vit C & zinc for wound healing. Vit K 10 mg IM q week if needed.
Trace elements zinc; copper; chromium; manganese, molybdenum, selenium.
May also add heparin, insulin, or albumin to PN solutions.

TIPS

Refeeding syndrome can occur in severely malnourished pts when refeeding begins at full kcal levels. May result in severely low levels of Mg²⁺, K⁺, Phos, fluid, & glucose. To prevent, begin feedings in these pts. at 75% BMR, then gradually ↑ to full kcal. Monitor Mg²⁺, K⁺, Phos, fluid, & glucose closely.
Minimum CHO's to prevent ketoacidosis is 100-150 g/day. >500 g/day CHO usually not tolerated (hyperglycemia, dehydration). Individual glucose oxidation rates ≈2-5 mg/kg/min.
Essential fatty acid depletion prevented by giving ≥500 cc 10% lipids twice weekly.
Max osmolarity is 900 mOsm; add 5 mg hydrocortisone if >600 mosm.
May cycle 16h/day to decrease risk of hepatic steatosis & increase anabolic production.
Monitor wt. changes, I/O's, FSBS q4-6h, Elect & BUN/Creat QD-QOD, SMA at least weekly once stable.
Contraindications to - Protein substrates: hypersensitivity, ↓blood vol, inborn errors of met, anuria.
Use special amino acid formulations for renal failure, severe liver dz, hepatic coma or encephalopathy.
Renal failure formulations: severe elect & acid-base imbalance, hyperammonemia.
Hepatic failure/Hepatic encephalopathy formulations: Anuria.
High metabolic stress formulations: Anuria, hyperammonemia, hepatic coma, severe elect & acid-base imbalance.
Complications - Catheter complications; Hepatic dysfunction, hyper & hypoglycemia, hyperosmolar nonketotic dehydration, fluid & elect imbalances (esp. phos & K⁺), metabolic acidosis, azotemia, infection, problems with line placement.

ENTERAL FORMULAS

	Kcal/ml	g protein/L	Nutrient base(ml)	Special features
Hepatic Aid	1.2	44.1	***	high-branch chain, low aromatic a.a.
Jevity	1.06	44.4	1321	isotonic, soluble fiber
Nepro	2.0	69.9	***	high cal, low fluid, low electrolytes
Pediasure	1.0	30.0	1000	isotonic, low residue, (1-6 yoa)
Perative	1.3	66.6	1155	high cal, protein, ß carotene & arginine for enhanced wound healing.
Pulmocare	1.5	62.6	947	low CHO, high fat, reduced CO₂
Suplena	2.0	30.0	***	high cal, low protein, fluid, & electrolytes
TwoCal HN	2.0	83.7	947	hyperosmolar, low residue
Vital HN	1.0	41.7	1500	elemental, low residue, free a.a. & peptides

MODULAR SUPPLEMENTS, PROTEIN

Gevral Protein (15.6 g protein, 7.05 g CHO, 52 mg fat, <50 mg Na⁺, ≥13 mg K⁺, 95.3 cal/26 g) 1/3 cup(≈26 g) in 8oz liquid. [8oz & 5lb containers]
Promod (5 g protein, 60 mg fat, 67 mg CHO, 44 mg Ca⁺⁺, 15 mg Na⁺, 65 mg K⁺, 33 mg Phos, 28 cal/6.6g scoop) 6.6 g powder to liquid, food, or enteral formula. [275 g cans]
Propac (3 g protein, 32 mg fat, 24 mg CHO, 14 mg Ca⁺⁺, 9 mg Na⁺, 20 mg K⁺, 12 mg Phos, 2 mg Mg⁺⁺, 16cal/4g) 1 tbsp(4 g) to liquid. [20 g packets, 350 g cans]

MODULAR SUPPLEMENTS, GLUCOSE POLYMERS

Polycose Liquid (50g CHO, 70mg Na⁺, 140mg Cl, 6mg K⁺, 20mg Ca²⁺, 3mg Phos, 200cal/100 ml) [126ml]
Polycose Powder (94g CHO, 110mg Na⁺, 223mg Cl, 10mg K⁺, 30mg Ca²⁺, 5mg Phos, 380cal/100g) [350g]
Moducal Powder (95g CHO, 70mg Na⁺, 150mg Cl, <10mg K⁺, 380cal/100 g) [368g]
Sumacal Powder (95g CHO, 100mg Na⁺, 210mg Cl, <39mg K⁺, 20mg Ca²⁺, <31mg Phos, 380cal/100g) [400g]

MODULAR SUPPLEMENTS, MISCELLANEOUS
<u>Lipomul</u> (10 g corn oil/15cc: 270 cal & 30 g fat/45 ml) [473 ml] 30-45 ml 2-4 times daily. *increases caloric intake*
<u>Microlipid</u> (50% fat emulsion of Safflower oil, polyglycerol esters of fatty acids, soy lecithin, xanthan gum, & ascorbic acid: 4500 cal & 500 g fat/liter) [120 ml] Supplies essential fatty acids & increase's calories.
<u>MCT</u> (lipid fraction of coconut oil containing medium chain triglycerides: 115 cal/15 ml) [quart] For pts who cannot digest & absorb conventional long chain fatty acids.

ORAL SUPPLEMENTS

	Kcal/8oz	g protein/8oz	Special features
<u>Choice DM</u>	250	10.6	low CHO with fiber for diabetics
<u>Ensure</u>	254	8.9	low residue
<u>Ensure Plus</u>	360	13.2	high cal, high protein, low residue
<u>Resource</u>	190	6.0/6oz	lactose free juice, protein fortified
<u>Sustacal</u>	242	14.6	high protein, low residue, lactose free
<u>Sustacal Plus</u>	365	14.6	high cal, high protein, low residue, lactose free
<u>Citrisource</u>	180	8.8	protein fortified clear liquid, low residue

PUDDINGS	Kcal/5oz	g protein/5oz	Special features
<u>Ensure</u>	250	6.8	low residue
<u>Sustacal</u>	240	6.8	low residue

MISCELLANEOUS
<u>alpha-αD-galactosidase</u> Enzyme [Beano] (liq, tab) use as directed
<u>Dairy Ease</u>] 1-3 tabs with first bite of dairy food
<u>lactase enzyme</u> *OTC*[Lactaid, Lactrase, Surelac]
<u>megestrol acetate</u> [Megace] (Susp 40 mg/ml) Anorexia: PO 800 mg/D
<u>orlistat</u> [Xenical] (Cap 120 mg) 120 mg with or within 1 hour after each meal. *Lipase inhibitor* ★

Nutrition Notes:

PRENATAL TESTING

- <10 wk.: transvaginal ultrasound can detect intrauterine pregnancy in 99% of cases when β-HCG > 1500 mlU/ml
- 10-12 wk.: Ultrasound for dating, PAP smear
- 14-18 wk.: Genetic testing if indicated,
- 15-20 wk.: Maternal α-fetoprotein, Hgb electrophoresis,
- 26-30 wk.: glucose tolerance test, UA, Rh & Indirect Coombs (RhoGAM?), Hct, Rubella titer.

ADMIT H & P

CC: Contractions (Ctx's) or spontaneous rupture of membranes (SROM)

Hx: Gravida( ); Para (Term, Preterm, Abortion, Living); FDLMP; EDC (by dates, US, exam); Gestation; Membrane status; Contraction pattern; Wt. gain; Complications during pregnancy.

Nagele's Rule: add 7 days to FDLMP, then count back 3 months.

Prenatal Lab: Rubella titer; Type & Rh; Indirect Coombs; Ultrasound; Other lab

Menstrual Hx: regular or not?; BCP use?

Medications, Allergies, Past Social Hx, Family Hx, ROS

EXAM: Vitals, Skin, HEENT, Heart, Lungs, edema, calf tenderness, neuro exam.

<u>Abdomen</u> - Fundal Height; Est. fetal weight; Fetal Heart Tones; Contraction rate & quality.

    <u>Pelvic</u> - Dilation (cm); Effacement (%) is the degree of shortening of cervical canal; Station (-3 to +3) is the distance between lowest bony portion of fetus and maternal ischial spines, Presenting part, Membrane status, Nitrazine (Ph of amniotic fluid is 7.1- 7.4), Ferning

Impression & Plan

LABOR

Contractions (Ctx's)

- True Labor: Ctx's occur at regular intervals; intervals gradually shorten; intensity gradually ↑s; discomfort in back & abd.; cervix dilates; Ctx's not stopped by sedation.
- False Labor: Ctx's at irregular intervals; intervals stay long; intensity stays unchanged; discomfort mainly in lower abd; cervix doesn't dilate; usually relieved by sedation.
- First Stage: Begins with effacement & dilatation

    latent - cervical change with regular Ctx's. First labor limit - 20.1 hr, avg. 6.4 hr; Second labor limit - 13.6hr, avg. 4.8 hr.

      • *active* - follows latent with rapid dilation; First labor limit - 11.7 hr, avg. 4.6 hr; Second labor limit - 5.2hr,avg 2.4 hr. Max dilatation >1.2 cm /hr (avg. 3 cm/hr); Max descent >1.0 cm/hr (avg. 3.3 cm/hr).

      • Second Stage: Begins with complete dilatation & ends with birth of baby; First labor limit - 2.9 hr., Second labor limit - 1.1 hr.

- Third Stage: Ends with delivery of the placenta.

FETAL ORIENTATION

- LOA - Left Occiput Anterior
- ROA - Right Occiput Anterior
- LOP - Left Occiput Posterior
- ROP - Right Occiput Posterior

FETAL MONITORING

- Baseline: normal 120-160 bpm's

    <120 is bradycardia

    >160 is tachycardia (DDX: prematurity, maternal fever, minimal fetal hypoxia, uterine tachysystole, drugs(atropine), arrhythmias, & hyperthyroidism.

- Variability:

    Long-Term Variability - An oscillation about the baseline at a frequency of 2-6 cycles/min with normal amplitude of 6-15 bpm.

    Short-Term Variability - Beat-to-beat changes in pulse rate from one moment to the next. Tracing looks "jiggly."

- Variable Decelerations - Possibly umbilical cord compression.

BPM	Duration (sec)		
	<30	30-60	≥60
>80	1	1	2
70-80	2	2	3
<70	2	3	4

(1)mild (2)moderate (3)moderate-severe (4)severe

- Late Decelerations - late onset, repetitive, & mirror Ctx's in symmetry. Associated with Uteroplacental insufficiency.

INTERVENTIONS
•Severe, prolonged variables: 1. change maternal position; 2. ↓ uterine activity (↓ oxytocin); 3. O₂; 4. Elevate presenting part; 5. Prepare for C-section
•Late Decelerations 1. Decrease uterine activity (↓ oxytocin); 2. Left lateral decubitus; 3. O₂; 4. Hydrate to expand blood volume; 5. Prepare for C-section

SCALP pH
  pH >7.2 = reassuring,   pH 7.2 - 7.25 = Pre-acidotic (repeat in 30 min)
  pH <7.2 = deliver promptly.

PAIN RELIEF Narcotics may be used generally if birth is anticipated within 1 - 2 hs. Remember they may prolong the latent phase & may depress a neonates respirations. A good combination is meperidine IV (rapid onset, short duration) & meperidine + Phenergan IM (slower onset, yet maintains blood levels longer).

ASSESSING CERVICAL RIPENESS:
THE BISHOP SCORE

DILATATION		EFFACEMENT		CONSISTENCY		CERVIX POSITION	
≤1 cm	0	≤40%	0	firm	0	posterior	0
1-2 cm	1	40-50%	1	medium	1	mid-position	1
3-4 cm	2	60-70%	2	soft	2	anterior	2
≥ 5 cm	3	≥80%	3				
	STATION						
≤-2	0	engaged	2				
2 to-1	1	≥+1	3				

A Bishop Score of ≥ 9 has a good prognosis for labor induction.

THE DELIVERY
Fetal orientation during labor & birth: engagement, flexion, descent, internal rotation, extension, external rotation, delivery of anterior shoulder, delivery of posterior shoulder.
Placenta should deliver within 20 min. First degree tear- break in skin or mucosa; Second degree tear extends into deeper tissues; Third degree tear- involves the anal sphincter; Fourth degree tear extends through anal sphincter and into the rectal mucosa.

ABNORMAL LABOR PATTERNS
Prolonged Latent Phase: Oxytocin & narcotic sedation can be effective therapies.
Protracted Active Phase: Ineffective Ctx's, large baby, small outlet, poorly positioned.
Arrested Active Phase: Oxytocin if problem with contractions; C-section if cephalopelvic disproportion.

THE APGAR SCORE

	0	1	2
Respiratory effort	None	Weak, irreg	Good, crying
Pulse	None	<100	>100
Muscle tone	Flaccid	↓ flexion	↑ flexion
Color	Pale blue	Body pink, Ext. blue	All pink
Reflex	None	Grimace	Cry, Irritability

APGAR ≥7: requires no assistance, APGAR 4-6: O₂ by flowby or assist with mask; stimulate by rubbing; assure newborn is warm & dry; monitor closely. APGAR ≤3: ABC's!!; establish IV & consider intubation; assess metabolic status & treat appropriately.

POSTPARTUM
Top of uterus is usually palpable at level of umbilicus
Lochia (vaginal discharge) usually does not exceed 1-2 pads/hr. The MC cause of excessive bleeding is uterine atony. Clots >50cc are abnormal.
Examine episiotomy if Pt. has fever or complains of pain over site.

THIRD TRIMESTER BLEEDING DDX
- Contact bleeding
- Cervical effacement & dilatation
- Placental abruption
- Cervical inflammation
- Placenta previa
- Cervical carcinoma or coagulation disorders

RhoGAM
RhoGAM (1cc vials of IgG anti-D given IM) Antepartum • *"micro-dose"* vial - protective for abortion, miscarriage, vaginal hemorrhage, ectopic pregnancy, or abdominal trauma occurring during the 1st 12 wk. of gestation. (protection against ≤2.5cc RBC's) • *standard dose Vial* - all unimmunized Rh(-) women receive around 28 wk. (protection against ≤15cc RBC's) • antepartum RhoGAM may cause (+) indirect Coombs in mother & does not indicate active immunization. Postpartum-1 standard dose vial is given within 72h of delivery to all RH(-) mothers delivering Rh(+) babies. Fetal screen testing on maternal blood will determine if fetal-maternal hemorrhage is >15cc, which requires >1 std dose vial of RhoGAM.

PRE-ECLAMPSIA
Risk factors: 1st pregnancy; extremes of age; multiple pregnancy.
Diagnosis of mild pre-eclampsia:
- *Hypertension* consisting of 1 of the following: Diastolic BP ≥90, Systolic ≥140, MAP ≥105, rise in systolic of 30, or rise of diastolic of 15.
- *Proteinuria* of >300 mg in 24 hr. Dipstick UA with ≥2+ protein is suspicious - recheck with cathed specimen.
- *Edema* - which is a non-specific finding in itself.
Diagnosis of severe pre-eclampsia: One of more of the following: Systolic ≥160;Diastolic ≥110;Oliguria (≤500cc/24h); Cyanosis; Pulmonary edema; Thrombocytopenia; IUGR; Proteinuria ≥5g/24h; Epigastric pain; Severe cerebral or visual disturbances
BP control: Usually treat DBP >105 with Hydralazine 5-10 mg IVP. This dose may be repeated in 15 minutes if no response is seen.

ECLAMPSIA
ECLAMPSIA is pre-eclampsia with the occurrence of a seizure not attributable to other causes. Seizure prophylaxis: 4-6 grams Magnesium Sulfate IVPB over 20 minutes, then continue at 2 grams/hr. Monitor DTR's (should diminish), clonus if present initially, respirations, & urine output frequently.

BREECH
- Frank Breech: presenting part is the buttocks, with legs flexed & parallel to thorax.
- Complete breech: presenting part is the buttocks, yet fetus is in a sitting position.
- Footling breech: presenting part is ≥1 foot.

TOCOLYSIS
TOCOLYSIS β_2 agonists: decreases smooth muscle tone in uterus, bronchioles, & vasculature. Side effects include: increased serum glucose, increased serum insulin, hypokalemia, decreased diastolic BP, increased maternal & fetal heart rate, tremor or jitteriness, seizures, pulmonary edema. **DRUGS**: *Ritodrine*. Magnesium sulfate: antagonizes Ca^{2+} in all muscle. At levels of 4 mEq/ml, DTR's are decreased; at 12 mEq/ml, respiratory depression & cardiac impairment ensues; between these two levels pt. will get flushing, HA, nystagmus, dysphoria.

MEDICATIONS
MEDICATIONS **Please refer to appropriate section for the dosage of a specific drug.
FDA Pregnancy category: A- adequate studies in pregnant women have not demonstrated a risk to the fetus in the first or later trimesters, B- animal studies have not demonstrated a risk to the fetus but there are no adequate studies in pregnant women or... animal studies have shown a adverse effect, but adequate studies in pregnant women have not demonstrated a risk to the fetus, C- animal studies have shown an adverse effect on the fetus but there are no adequate studies in humans; the benefits from the use of the drug may be acceptable despite its potential risks, or there are no animal or human studies, D- there is evidence of human fetal risk, but the potential benefits from the use of the drug may be acceptable despite its potential risks, X- studies have demonstrated fetal abnormalities or adverse reaction reports indicate evidence of fetal risk, the risk clearly outweighs any possible benefit.
KEY- A, B, C, D, X = pregnancy category; Lactation-☒= unsafe;?= questionable or not known; ☑= felt to be safe
ANALGESICS: acetaminophen- A,☑; aspirin- D,?; codeine- C,?; diclofenac- B,☒; ibuprofen- D in 3rd ,B in 1st & 2nd,☑; ketoprofen-B,☒; naproxen- B,☒;meperidine- C,?; methadone- C,?; propoxyphene- C,?; salicylates- D,?; tolmetin- C,☒.
ANTICOAGULANTS: aspirin- D; Coumadin- X; heparin- C

<u>ANTIMICROBIALS</u>: acyclovir- C,?; azithromycin- B,? ; cephalosporins- B,?; chloramphenicol- C,☒
;clotrimazole- B,?; erythromycin- B,☑; erythromycin estolate-B elevated LFT in 10% cases, ☑; gentamicin-
D,?; isoniazid- C,?; lindane- B,?; metronidazole- 1ˢᵗ trimester B, ?; nitrofurantoin- B,☑; nystatin- A,?;
penicillins- B,?; sulfonamides- C,☒; tetracycline- D,☒; triamcinolone intranasal- C,?;trimethoprim-C,☒.

<u>ENDOCRINE</u>: insulin- B,☑

<u>ENT</u>: beclomethasone intranasal- C,?; brompheniramine- C,☒; dexamethasone intranasal-
C,☒;dextromethorphan- ?,?; diphenhydramine- B,☒; pseudoephedrine- C,☒; terfenadine- C,☒

<u>GI</u>: antacids- generally accepted after 1ˢᵗ trimester,?; bisacodyl- ?,?; cimetidine- B, ?; docusate- AC, droperidol-
generally accepted,?; famotidine- B, ?; prochlorperazine- C, ?; psyllium- generally accepted,?; AC, ranitidine-
B,?; simethicone- C,?; trimethobenzamide- AC.

<u>NEUROLOGIC</u>: carbamazepine- C, ?; ergotamine- X,?; phenobarbital- D, ?; phenytoin- D,?; valproic acid- D,?

<u>PULMONARY</u>: albuterol-C,?; epinephrine-C,☒; inhaled steroids-C,D,☒; steroids oral-C, ☒, terbutaline-B,☒;
theophylline-C, ?

<u>PSYCHIATRIC</u>: benzodiazepines- X&D, ☒; fluoxetine C,?; haloperidol- C,?; hydroxyzine- C,☒; lithium- D,☒;
phenothiazine- C,D,?; sertraline-C, ?; tricyclics- C,D,?.

OTHER OB MEDS

<u>ergonovine</u> [Ergotrate] (Tab 0.2m g) IM 0.2 mg or PO 0.2-0.4 mg q6-8h prn

<u>magnesium sulfate</u> (Sol 10-20%) eclampsia- IV 1-4 g over 2-4, titrate drip to reflexes 5 g in 250ml D5W (20
mg/ml) at 1g/h (50 ml/h)

<u>methylergonovine</u> [Methergine] (Tab 0.2 mg) PO/IM 0.2 mg q 6h prn

<u>oxytocin</u> [Pitocin] IM 10 units after delivery of placenta, postpartum hemorrhage- IV 10-40units in 1000 ml NS

<u>RHO immune globulin</u> [RhoGam] IM 1 vial within 72h of delivery if mother Rh neg

<u>ritodrine</u> [Yutopar] (Tab 10 mg) IV 150 mg in 500ml D5W (0.3 mg/ml) at 0.1-0.35 mg/min (24-83 ml/h), PO 10-20
mg q 4h

OB Notes:

ANESTHETICS
proparacaine [Ophthaine, Ophthetic] (0.5%) 1 drop q5-10 minutes; MAX 5-7 doses
tetracaine [Pontacaine HCl] (Sol & oint 0.5%) 1-2 drop or 0.5-1 inch ointment

ANTI-INFECTIVES
bacitracin ointment q3-4h
bacitracin + polymyxin [Polysporin] ointment q3-4h
bacitracin+neomycin+polymyxin [Neosporin] ointment q3-4h, drop q1-6h
chloramphenicol [Chloromycetin] 1% ointment q3-4h
ciprofloxacin [Ciloxan] (0.3% drop) 1drop q2h while awake for 2 days, then 1drop q4h while awake for 5 days
Cortisporin [polymyxin B/neomycin/hydrocortisone] 1-2 drop TID/QID
erythromycin [Ilotycin] (0.5% oint) QD or more
gentamicin [Garamycin] (0.3%) oint TID/QID, 2 drop q1h
norfloxacin [Chibroxin] (0.3%) 1-2 drop QID for up to 7 days
ofloxacin [Ocuflox] (0.3%) 1-2 drop q3-4h
sulfacetamide [Sulamyd] (10, 30%) 1-2 drop q2-3h, (10%) Oint BID/QID
sulfacetamide + prednisolone [Metimyd] (10%/0.5%) oint TID/QID, 2-3 drop q1-2h
tetracycline [Achromycin] (1%) oint q3-4h, 2 drop q1-6h
tobramycin [Tobrex] (0.3%) oint q3-4h, drop q1-6h
trifluridine [Viroptic] (1%) 1 drop q2h while awake
vidarabine [Vira-A] (3%) 0.5 inch oint five times a day

GLAUCOMA AGENTS (Sym- sympathomimetic; β- Beta blocker; DM- direct miotics; CI- Carbonic Anhydrase Inhibitors)
betaxolol HCl [Betopic, Betoptic S] β (susp 0.25, sol 0.5%) 1 drop BID
brimonidine [Alphagan] (sol 0.2%) 1 drop in affected eye(s) TID (≈8h apart). (5 or 10ml dropper bottle)
brinzolamide [Azopt] CI (sol 1%, 2.5, 5, 10, 15 ml Drop-Tainers) One drop in the affected eye TID
carteolol [Ocupress] β (sol 1%) 1 drop BID
Cosopt [dorzolamide 2%/ timolol 0.5%] CI/β(sol 5, 10 ml ocumeters) One drop in the affected eye BID
demecarium bromide [Humorsol] CI (sol 0.125, 0.25%) 1-2 drops twice a week up to 2 drops BID
dipivefrin [Propine] Sym (sol 0.1%) 1 drop q12h
epinephrine HCl [Epifrin] Sym (sol 0.1, 0.25, 0.5, 1, 2%) 1-2 drops QD/BID
isoflurophate [Floropryl] CI (gel 0.025%) 0.25 inch q8-72h
latanoprost [Xalatan] (Sol 0.005%, 50mcg/ml) glaucoma 1 drop in affected eye once a day.
levobunolol HCl [Betagan Liquifilm] β (sol 0.25, 0.5%) 1 drop QD/BID
metipranolol HCl [OptiPranolol] β (sol 0.3%) 1 drop BID
physostigmine [Isopto Eserine] CI (sol 0.25%) 2 drops up to 4 times daily
pilocarpine [Pilocar, Isopto Carpine] DM (sol 0.25, 0.5, 1, 2, 4, 6, 8, 10%) 1-2 drops up to 6 times daily
timolol maleate [Timoptic, Timoptic XE] β (sol 0.25, XE- Gel sol 0.5%) 1 drop BID, XE 1 drop QD

MYDRIATICS/ VASOCONSTRICTORS/ CYCLOPLEGICS
atropine sulfate [Isopto atropine] (0.5, 1, 2, 3%) 1-2 drops up to QID. Cycloplegia and mydriasis 7-14d
cyclopentolate [Cyclogyl] (0.5, 1, 2%) 1 drop; cycloplegia and mydriasis may last up to 24h
homatropine [Isopto Homatropine] (2, 5%) 1-2 drops q3-4h; cycloplegia and mydriasis 1-3d
hydroxyamphetamine [Paredrine] (1%) 1-2 drops; mydriasis may persist up to 3h
phenylephrine HCl [Neo Synephrine] (2.5,10%) 1 drop solution; mydriasis may persist up to 7h; No cycloplegia
scopolamine [Isopto Hyoscine] (0.25%) 1-2 drops up to QID; cycloplegia and mydriasis may last 3-7 days
tropicamide [Mydriacyl] (0.5, 1%) 1-2 drops; cycloplegia and mydriasis may last 6h

STEROIDS
dexamethasone [Decadron] (drop 0.1%; oint 0.05%) 1-2 drops q1h daytime & q2h night then 1-2 drop q4-8h as eye improves; oint thin film TID/QID
fluorometholone [Flarex] (Susp 0.1%) 1-2 drops QID; May start with 2 drops q2° for first 24-48°
fluorometholone [FML, FML Forte] (0.25% Susp; 0.1% Oint) 1 drop BID/TID or ointment 1-3 times daily
loteprednol [Lotemax 0.5%-2.5, 5, 10, 15 ml] (0.5% drops); [Alrex 0.2%- 5, 10 ml ocumeters] One drop QID
medrysone [HMS] (Susp 1%) 1 drop up to every 4 hours
Pred mild [prednisolone] (Susp 0.12%) 2 drops q1° for 24-48h, then 1-2 drop 2-4 times/day. *Sulfites*
prednisolone [Pred Forte] (1% drops) 2 drops q1° for 24-48°, then 1-2 drop 2-4 times/day. *Contains sulfites*
rimexolone [Vexol] (Susp 1%) *Anterior uveitis* 1-2 drops q1h while awake 1st wk, then 1 drop q2h 2nd wk, then taper; *Post op* 1-2 drops QID X 2wks

MISC AGENTS (AH – antihistamine; MSS – mast cell stabilizer; VC - vasoconstrictor)

<u>artificial tears</u> [Lacril, Tears Naturale, Tears Plus] 1-2 drops prn

<u>cromolyn</u> [Crolom] (Sol 4%) *>4yoa* 1-2 drops each eye 4-6 times daily. MSS

<u>emedastine</u> [Emadine] (Sol 0.05%)One drop to QID prn allergic conjunctivitis

<u>fluorescein sodium</u> [Fluor-I-Strip] (strip 0.6, 1, 9 mg; sol 2%) 1-2 drops to stain eye

<u>ketorolac</u> [Acular] (Sol 0.5%) 1 drop QID. NSAID

<u>ketotifen</u> [Zaditor] (Sol 0.025%) 1 drop in affected eye q8-12 hrs. (5, 7.5 ml) *allergic conjunctivitis* ★

<u>levocabastine</u> [Livostin] (Susp 0.05%) *Adults* 1 drop QID. AH

<u>lodoxamide</u> [Alomide] (Sol 0.1%) *>2yoa* 1-2 drops QID up to 3 months. MSS

<u>Naphcon A</u> [naphazoline 0.025% + pheniramine 0.3%] *>6yoa* 1-2 drops up to QID. AH, VC

<u>olopatadine</u> [Patanol] (Sol 0.1%) *>3yoa use* 1-2 drops in affected eye q6-8*. MSS

Ophthalmology Notes:

ABC's and O_2 before Drugs!

AGE	WEIGHT	DEFIB	ET TUBE	EPINEPHRINE	LIDOCAINE	ATROPINE	BRETYLIUM	BICARBONATE	NARCAN	MANNITOL	DEXTROSE 50	FUROSEMIDE	CaCl 10%	ALBUTEROL	TERBUTALINE	PHENYTOIN	DIAZEPAM
Unit	KG	J	Mm	mg	mg	mg	Mg	Meq	mg	gm	ml	ml	ml	ml	mg	mg	mg
Dose Unit/kg		2		.01	1.0	.02	5.0	1.0	0.1	.25-2	1-2	1-2	0.3		.01	15	0.2
Route				IV	IV	IV	IV	IV	IV	IV	IV	IV	IV	Aerosol		IV	
Freq	min			5	5-8	5	5	10	2-3								15	2-5
PRE	2	4	2.5	.02	2.0	0.1	10	3.0	0.2	2.0	2.0	2.0	0.6	.25	.02	30	0.4
NB	3.5	7	3.0	.04	3.5	0.1	18	5.0	0.4	3.5	3.5	3.5	1.1	.25	.04	53	0.7
2m	5	10	3.5	.05	5.0	0.1	25	5.0	0.5	5.0	5.0	5.0	1.5	.25	.05	75	1.0
4m	6.5	13	3.5	.07	6.5	.14	32	5.0	0.7	6.5	6.5	6.5	2.0	.25	.07	98	1.3
6m	8	16	3.5	.08	8.0	.16	40	5.0	0.8	8.0	8.0	8.0	2.4	.25	.08	120	1.6
9m	9	18	4.0	.09	9.0	.18	45	5.0	0.9	9.0	9.0	9.0	2.7	.25	.09	135	1.8
1y	10	20	4.0	.10	10	0.2	50	10	1.0	10	10	10	3.0	0.5	0.1	150	2.0
2y	13	26	4.5	.13	11	.26	65	13	1.3	13	13	13	3.9	0.5	.13	195	2.6
4y	17	35	4.5	.17	17	.34	85	15	1.7	17	17	17	5.1	0.5	.17	255	3.4
6y	20	45	5.0	.21	21	.42	100	20	2.1	20	20	20	6.0	0.5	.20	300	4.0
8y	25	50	5.5	.25	25	.50	125	25	2.5	25	25	25	7.5	0.5	.25	375	5.0
10y	30	55	6.0	.30	30	.60	140	30	3.0	30	30	30	9.0	0.5	0.3	450	6.0
12y	35	65	6.5	.35	35	.70	160	35	3.5	35	35	35	11	0.5	.35	525	7.0
14y	40	85	7.0	0.4	40	0.8	180	45	4.0	40	40	40	12	0.5	0.4	600	8.0
16y	45	95	7.0	.45	45	0.9	200	50	4.5	45	45	45	14	0.5	.45	675	9.0

FLUIDS & ELECTROLYTES

MAINTENANCE REQUIREMENTS
100 cc/kg/24hr for the 1st 10kg
50 cc/kg/24hr for the 2nd 10kg
20 cc/kg/24hr for after 20kg

DEHYDRATION: Signs & Symptoms
MILD -5% thirsty, restless
MODERATE -10% thirsty, irritable or lethargic, dry mucosa, tachycardia, ↓ tears, ↓ fontanel, ↓ urine output, deep respirations
SEVERE -15% impending shock, drowsy, cold, limp, peripheral cyanosis, tachycardia, tachypnea, sunken fontanel, no tears, anuria, ↓ BP

IV FLUIDS	mEq/L Na⁺	Cl	Glu
D5¼ Normal Saline 0.2%	38	38	50gm
D5½ Normal Saline 0.45%	77	77	50gm
Normal Saline - 0.9%	154	154	

Volume Deficit = Wt(kg) x 10 x % dehydration

ORAL REHYDRATION Mild - 50 ml/kg/4hr, 100ml/kg/24hr
Moderate - 100 ml/kg/6hr then 100 ml/kg/24hr
IV REHYDRATION- Determine Na⁺ & H₂O deficits. Initial therapy: Rapid re-expansion of ECF until stable with isotonic saline or lactated ringers in 20-30 ml/kg challenges, may repeat twice if needed. If repeat boluses not successful may require 10ml/kg blood. Subsequent Therapy: Replace remaining deficit as outlined below when hemodynamically stable.

CLASSES OF DEHYDRATION	FLUID CORRECTION
Hypotonic (Na⁺ < 130 mEq/L) → → →	Rapid ↑ Na⁺ to 120 mEq/L, ↑ to 130 over 24-36hr
Isotonic (Na⁺ 130-150 mEq/L) → → →	Replace ½ over 12hr; then ¼ over 12hr twice
Hypertonic (Na⁺ > 150 mEq/L) → → →	Slowly ↓ Na⁺ 10 mEq/L/24hr over 36-48hr

Na⁺ Correction =[desired- measured] x [Wt x 0.6]

LANE = Drugs down the ET tube: Lidocaine, Atropine, Naloxone, and Epinephrine
ET tube size (mm) = [16 + Age (yrs)] ÷ 4

IV Drips	mcg/kg/min	Dilution in 100cc D₅W	Infusion Rate 1 cc/hr =
Lidocaine	20-50	6.0 mg/kg	1.0 mcg/kg/min
Epinephrine	0.1-1.0	0.6 mg/kg	0.1 mcg/kg/min
Dopamine	2-20	6.0 mg/kg	1.0 mcg/kg/min
Dobutamine	5-20	6.0 mg/kg	1.0 mcg/kg/min

$$\text{IV Infusions:} \quad \frac{\text{mg Drug}}{100\text{cc Fluid}} = 6 \times \frac{\text{Desired dose (mcg/kg/min) x Wt(kg)}}{\text{Desired rate (cc/hr)}}$$

Basic Life Support		
BLS Steps	Infant (0 -1 yr)	Child (1 - 8yr)
Assess Responsiveness	Gently tap and speak loudly	
Call for Help		
Position	Supine on firm surface	
Open Airway	Head tilt/chin lift if no trauma or Jaw Thrust if trauma suspected	
Look, Listen & Feel for Respiration		
Two Breaths (1-1.5 sec/breath) if no spontaneous respirations. If not effective reposition and retry, if still ineffective check for FBAO.		
Check Pulse	Brachial	Carotid
Activate EMS- Lone rescuer should perform BLS for 1min before leaving to activate EMS. May move patient if no trauma.		
Compression Position Lower 1/3 sternum	2-3 Fingers	Heel of one hand
Compression Depth	0.5-1.0 inch	1.0-1.5 inch
Compression Rate	>100/min	>100/min
Compression/Ventilation	5 to 1	5 to 1
Ventilation Rate	20/min (1 q3 sec)	20/min (1 q3 sec)
FBAO - CONSCIOUS, WITNESSED		
Assess airway: Listen, Tongue & Jaw Lift	Attempt to clear airway if witnessed or unable to perform rescue breathing. Encourage spontaneous coughing. Intervene if cough ineffective or if patient becomes unconscious	
Maneuver	5 Back blows, then 5 Chest thrusts	3-5 Abdominal thrusts
Head tilt/chin lift, remove foreign body if visible (no blind finger sweeps). Attempt rescue breaths, repeat maneuvers until obstruction is cleared.		

PEDIATRIC ANALGESICS / SEDATIVES

acetaminophen [Tylenol] (Chw 80, 160 mg; Drp 80 mg/0.8cc; Elx 160 mg/5cc; Liq 500 mg/15cc; Syp 160 mg/5cc; Supp 120, 325 & 650 mg) PO 10-15 mg/kg q4-6h. Supp PR >6yr 325mg q4-6h, 3-6yr 120mg q4-6h PRN pain/fever *Contraindicated in G6PD Deficiency!

chloral hydrate [Noctec] (Tab 250, 500 mg; Elx 250, 500 mg/5cc; Supp 324, 500, 648 mg) PO 25-50 mg/kg, MAX 2g, may repeat 25 mg/kg in 30min if 1st dose ineffective.

diazepam [Valium] PO 0.2-0.5 mg/kg; IV 0.1-0.2 mg/kg q2-4h

ibuprofen [Children's Advil, Children's Motrin] (elixir 100mg/5ml) PO 5-10 mg/kg q4-6h prn

meperidine (C2) [Demerol] IM 1-1.5 mg/kg q3-4h prn; MAX 100 mg

midazolam C4 [Versed] Pediatric dose for sedation, anxiolysis, or amnesia: 0.1-0.15 mg/kg IM, may use up to 0.5 mg/kg not to exceed 10 mg.

morphine sulfate (C2) 0.1-0.2 mg/kg IM, IV, SQ q1-4h, MAX 15 mg/dose

PEDIATRIC ANTIHISTAMINE / DECONGESTANTS

chlorpheniramine maleate PO 0.35 mg/kg/24h ÷q4-6h; SR PO 0.2 mg/kg/24h ÷q12h; MAX 24 mg/24h

cetirizine [Zyrtec] (Tabs 5, 10 mg; Syrup 1 mg/ml) 2-5 yoa 2.5-5ml QD or 2.5ml BID; ≥6yoa 5-10 mg QD★

diphenhydramine [Benadryl] PO/IM/IV 5 mg/kg/24h ÷q6h; MAX 300 mg/24h

loratadine [Claritin] (Tabs & Redi tabs 10 mg; Syr 1 mg/ml) >6yrs 10 mg QD★

Phenergan Syrup Plain (promethazine 6.25 mg & ETOH 7%/5cc) PO 2-6y 1.25cc q4-6h; 6-12y 2.5cc q4-6h; >12y 5.0cc q4-6h

Phenergan with codeine (promethazine 6.25 mg, ETOH 7% & Codeine 10 mg/5cc) Dose as above.

Phenergan with dextromethorphan (promethazine 6.25 mg, ETOH 7% & DM 15 mg /5cc) Dose as above.

<u>Rondec DM Oral Drops</u> {& Syrup} (pseudoephedrine 25 mg {60 mg}, DM 15 mg {15 mg}, carbinoxamine 2 mg {4 mg} /ml {5ml}). Oral Drops: *1-3 mo* ¼ ml QID, *3-6 mo* ½ ml QID, *6-9 mo* ¾ ml QID; *9-18 mo* 1 ml; Syrup: *18 mo -6y* 2.5 ml QID, *>6y* 5 ml QID

PEDIATRIC ANTIMICROBIALS

PEDIATRIC FEVERS: DDX: Meningitis, Pneumonia, OM, Sepsis, UTI, Joints, Epiglottitis, Infective diarrhea/Abd infection, viral, endocarditis.

age <2-3 months, rectal temp >100.4°F; Most common bacterial organisms: group B streptococcus, enterics, H. influenza, pneumococcus. Consider viral pathogens: CMV and HSV. History of maternal STD, perinatal fever, chorioamnionitis, fussiness, poor feeding, decreased activity. Septic work up: CBC, blood culture, UA, urine culture, Urine CIE, CXR, Lumbar puncture [#1 C&S, gram stain; #2 glucose, protein, Well-Cogens (H. Inf, N. gonorrhea); #3 cell count]. Treatment- admit all infants < 28 days old with temp >100.4° for IV antibiotics until cultures proven negative at 48 hours. Infants 29-60 days of age may warrant admission depending on findings or if unremarkable workup may be given ceftriaxone IM 100 mg/kg and followed up at 24 hours.

age 3-36 months with rectal temperature greater than 103° F without a source deserve a workup including- history and physical, urine analysis, urine and blood cultures, CBC. Consider performing a lumbar puncture. Treatment- amoxicillin 80 mg/kg divided TID or ceftriaxone IM 100 mg/kg divided Q 12 hours- pending cultures. Positive cultures warrant a 10-day course of treatment. Admit for IV antibiotic if remains febrile or otherwise clinically indicated. Always follow up by phone or in clinic.

Treat source of fever when found. Lower temp acetaminophen or ibuprofen.

PEDIATRIC SEPSIS

Patient	Neonate <4 days	>5 days	Child
Common Organisms	Group B strep, E. Coli, Klebsiella, Enterobacteriaceae, Staph aureus, Listeria monocytogenes	Haemophilus influenza, Group B strep, E. Coli, Klebsiella, Enterobacteriaceae, Staph aureus, Listeria monocytogenes	Strep pneumonia, Haemophilus influenza, Meningococci, Staph aureus
Empiric Antibiotic	Ampicillin & cefotaxime	Ampicillin & cefotaxime or ceftriaxone	cefuroxime, cefotaxime or ceftriaxone

Adapted from Guide to Antimicrobial Therapy, 1997, p.43

<u>acyclovir</u> [Zovirax] (Tab 400, 800; Cap 200 mg; Elx 200 mg/ml) Neonate: *Herpes Simplex,* 10 mg/kg q8h. Children: *Mucocutaneous* PO 250 mg/kg/24h ÷q8h; *Encephalitis* PO 10 mg/kg ÷q8h.
<u>acyclovir sodium</u> [Zovirax for IV only] (500 mg per 10ml vials, 1000 mg per 20ml vials) For children under 12 yoa: *Mucosal & Cutaneous HSV in immunocompromised Pts* - 250 mg/m² IV over 1h q8h X 7D; *Herpes Simplex Encephalitis & Varicella Zoster in immunocompromised Pts* - 500 mg/m² over 1h q8h X7D.
<u>amoxicillin</u> [Amoxil] (Tab 125, 250, 500; Elx 125 & 250 mg/5ml) PO 20-40 mg/kg/24 ÷q8h; OM prophylaxis 20 mg/kg/24h ÷q12h
<u>amoxicillin clavulanate</u> [Augmentin] (Chw 125, 200, 250, 400; Elx 125, 200, 250, 400 mg/5ml, Tab 250, 500) PO 20*- 40**mg/kg/24h ÷q8h; 25* or 45**mg/kg/24h ÷ q12h. *less severe infections. **OM, lower resp, Sin, severe infections★
<u>ampicillin</u> [Principen] (Tab 125, 250 & 500 mg; IM/IV 125, 250 & 500 mg,1 & 2g) PO <2kg 50 mg/kg/24h ÷q12h; >2kg 100 mg/kg/24h ÷q12h; <40kg 50-100 mg/kg/24h ÷q6h; *Severe infect* 150-300 mg/kg/24h; >40kg 150-300 mg/kg/24h ÷q6h; *Severe infect* 250-500 mg/kg/24h
<u>azithromycin</u> [Zithromax] (Susp 125, 250mg/5ml) PO phar (>2 yr old)- 12mg/kg qD for 5 days; OM (>6 months old)- 10mg/kg PO day 1, then 5mg/kg PO days 2- 5★
<u>cefaclor</u> [Ceclor] (Caps 250, 500; Elx 125, 187, 250 & 375 mg/5ml) PO 20-40 mg/kg/24h ÷q8h
<u>cefadroxil</u> [Duricef, Ultracef] (Caps 500; Elx 125, 250, 500 mg/5ml) PO 30 mg/kg/24h ÷q12h
<u>cefamandole</u> [Mandol] (Vials 500mg, 1, 2 gm) 50-100mg/kg/24h IM/IV ÷ q4-8h★
<u>cefazolin</u> [Kefzol, Ancef] (Vial 500 mg & 1 gm) IV/IM 25-100 mg/kg/24h ÷ q6h or 8h★
<u>cefixime</u> [Suprax] (Tab 200, 400 mg; Susp 100 mg/5cc) 8 mg/kg/24h PO dosed QD or BID★
<u>cefotaxime</u> [Claforan] IM/IV 50-200 mg/kg/24h ÷q-4-6h★
<u>cefpodoxime</u> [Vantin] (Tab 100, 200 mg; Susp 50, 100 mg/5cc) 10 mg/kg/24h PO ÷ 12h★
<u>cefprozil</u> [Cefzil] PO *Otitis Media* 30 mg/kg/24h ÷q12h; *Pharyngitis* 15 mg/kg/24h ÷q12h
<u>ceftizoxime</u> [Cefizox] 50 mg/kg/dose IV/IM q6-8h★
<u>ceftriaxone</u> [Rocephin] IM/IV 50-75 mg/kg/24h ÷q12-24h; *Meningitis* IV 100 mg/kg/day ÷q12h. MAX 4g/24h.
<u>cefuroxime</u> [Zinacef, Ceftin] *Neonate* IM/IV 20-40 mg/kg/24h ÷q12h. *Infant/Child* IM/IV 50-100 mg/kg/24h ÷q6-8h. *Meningitis* IV 200-240 mg/kg/24h ★
<u>cephalexin</u> [Keflex] (Caps 250, 500; Elx 125, 250 mg/5ml) PO 20-50 mg/kg/24h ÷q6h
<u>clarithromycin</u> [Biaxin] (Susp 125 & 250mg/5ml;Tab 250, 500mg) PO 7.5mg/kg BID★

clindamycin [Cleocin] (Tab 75, 150; Elx 75 mg/5ml) *Neonate* IM/IV 15 mg/kg/24h ÷q8h. *Children* PO 10-20 mg/kg/24h ÷q6-8h; IV/IM 15-40 mg/kg/24h ÷q6-8h

cloxacillin [Cloxapen, Tegopen] (Cap 250, 500mg; Susp 125mg/5cc) PO 50-100mg/kg/24h÷q6h★

dicloxacillin [Dycill, Dynapen, Pathocil] (Cap 125, 250, 500mg; Susp 62.5mg/5cc) PO <40kg 12.5-25 mg/kg/24h ÷ q6h, >40kg 125-250mg q6h. Not recommended for newborns★

erythromycin estolate [Ilosone] (Tab 250, 500mg; Susp 125, 250mg/5cc) 30-50 mg/kg PO ÷ q6 or 12h★

erythromycin ethyl succinate [EES] (Tab 200,400mg;Elx 200,400mg/5ml;Drp50mg/5ml)PO 30-50mg/kg/24h ÷q6h

erythromycin lactobionate (Vial 500mg, 1 gm) 15-20 mg/kg/24h IV ÷ q6h (4 grams/24h max)★

loracarbef [Lorabid] (Susp 100, 200 mg/5cc, Tab 200, 400 mg) *6 mos-12 yrs* use 15-30 mg/kg/24h PO ÷ q12h★

nafcillin [Nafcil, Unipen, Nallpen] (Vials 500mg, 1, 2gm; Cap250mg; Tab 500mg; Susp 250mg/5cc) IM 25 mg/kg BID or IV/IM 100-200mg/kg/24h divided in 4-6 doses; PO 25-50mg/kg/24h ÷ QID★

oxacillin [Bactocill, Prostaphlin] (Vials 250, 500mg, 1, 2, 4 gm; Cap 250, 500mg; Sol 250mg/5cc) IV/IM:<40lbs use 50-100 mg/kg/24h IV/IM ÷ q6h. PO:<40lbs use 50-100 mg/kg/24h PO ÷ q6h★

Pediazole [200mg erythromycin ethylsuccinate + 600mg sulfisoxazole per 5cc] 50 mg/kg/24h based on erythromycin component, OR 150 mg/kg/24h based on sulfa component, ÷ equally q6 or 8h★

penicillin G benzathine [Bicillin] (IM 0.3,0.6 millionU) *congenital syphilis* IM 50,000 U/kg; *Grp A&B Strep* IM 0.6-1.2 millionU

penicillin G *Neonates* IM/IV 0.05-0.1 millionU/kg/24h ÷q12h. *Group B Strep meng* IM/IV 240,000 U/kg/24h ÷q8h

penicillin V potassium [Pen Vee K, Ledercillin VK] (250, 500 mg tablets; 125, 250 mg/5cc suspension; 400,000 units = 250mg) 25-50 mg/kg/24h ÷ q6-8h. (acid stable)★

trimethoprim/sulfamethoxazole (TMP/SMX) [Bactrim, Septra] PO 8 mg TMP/kg/24h ÷q12h. (1 ml susp/kg/day). IV 8-10 mg/kg/24h ÷q12h

PEDIATRIC CARDIOLOGY

atropine .02 mg/kg IV q2-5 min.

Defibrillation 2 Joules/kg.

digoxin for CHF (increase dose for SVT). Total Digitalizing Dose (TDD): give 1/2 TDD initially, then 1/4 TDD q8-18h x 2 doses. Maintenance Dose (MD): <10y bid, >10y q day. Dose unit mcg/kg.

Age	PO TDD	IV/IM TDD	PO MD	IV/IM MD
Prem	20	15	5	3-4
Term	30	20	8-10	6-8
<2yr	40-50	30-40	10-12	7.5-9
2-10y	30-40	20-30	8-10	6-8
>10y	.75-1.25 mg		0.125-.25 mg	

epinephrine (1:10,000) *Bradycardia/hypotension* IV 0.01 mg/kg q3-5 min. MAX 0.5 mg

lidocaine IV 1.0 mg/kg q5-8 min prn. MAX 3 mg/kg. 20-50 mcg/kg/min IV drip

PEDIATRIC DRUG OVERDOSES

charcoal PO 15-30 grams. If it contains sorbitol, no cathartic is needed. If not, use: magnesium citrate 4cc/kg (MAX 200cc)

naloxone [Narcan] (0.2, 0.4 & 1.0 mg/ml) IM/IV 5-10 mcg/kg/dose q3-5 min prn. MAX 2 mg.

PEDIATRIC NEUROLOGY

carbamazepine [Tegretol] (Chw 100 & 200 mg; Susp 100 mg/5ml) PO 10 mg/kg/24h ÷q12h. MAX: *<6y* 20 mg/kg/24h, *6-12y* 100 mg/kg/24h. Serum Concentration 4-12 mg/L.

phenobarbital [Luminal] (Tab 15, 30 & 60 mg; Elx 3 & 4 mg/ml; Inj 30, 60, 65 & 130 mg/ml) *epilepsy*; Loading dose (IV): *Neonate:* 15-20 mg/kg; *Inf/Child/Adolescent:* 15-18 mg/kg; MAX: 30 mg/kg. Maintenance dose (IV, PO): QD or ÷BID dosing: *Neonate:* 3-5 mg/kg/24h; *Infant:* 5-6 mg/kg/24h; *1-5y:* 6-8 mg/kg/24h; *6-12y:* 4-6 mg/kg/24h; *Adolescent:* 1-3 mg/kg/24h; MAX: 1-2 gm. Serum level 15-40 mg/L

phenytoin [Dilantin] *Status epilepticus:* IV 15-20 mg/kg. Maint dose (PO, IV) 5 mg/kg/24h ÷q8-12h; *Inf/child:* 5 mg/kg/24h ÷q8-12h. Serum Level 10-20 mg/L

primidone [Mysoline] (Tabs 50 & 250 mg; Susp 50 mg/ml) PO 10-25 mg/kg/24h ÷q6-8h

PEDIATRIC PULMONOLOGY

albuterol [Proventil] (MDI; Syrup 2 mg/5ml; Tab 2,4 mg) MDI: 1-2 inhalations q4-6h. Nebulizer: 0.01-0.03ml/kg (1ml max) of 5 mg/ml soln in 2.5 ml of NS q20-30 min; PO: *2-5 yr-* 0.3 mg/kg q8h. *6-11 yr-* 2 mg ÷ q6-8h (max 24 mg/24h) *>12 yr-* 2-4 mg PO TID or QID (max 8 mg QID)

aminophylline [Somophyllin] IV Loading Dose: 6 mg/kg over 20 min. Maintenance Dose:(Continuous IV drip) *Neonate:* 0.2 mg/kg/hr; *1mo-1yr:* 0.2-0.9 mg/kg/hr; *1-9yr:* 1.0 mg/kg/hr; *>9yr:* 0.8 mg/kg/hours

calfactant [Infasurf] lung surfactant for prevention and treatment of RDS in premature infants. Intratracheal suspension 3 ml/kg body wt at birth, every 12 hours, up to 3 doses

montelukast [Singulair] (Chew 5 mg, Tab 10mg) PO 6-14 yrs 5 mg Q evening; >14 yr 10 mg QD **(leukotriene inhibitor)**★

<u>prednisone</u> *Asthma exacerbation*: 0.5-2 mg/kg/24h up to 20-40 mg/24h x 3-5 days.

<u>theophylline</u> Loading Dose: 0.8 mg/kg/dose to ↑ serum theophylline level by 2 mg/L. Maintenance Dose (PO): *0-2 mo:* 3-6 mg/kg/24h ÷q8h; *2-6 mo:* 6-15 mg/kg/24hr ÷q6hr; *6-12 mo:* 15-22 mg/kg/24hr ÷q4-6h; *1-9y:* 22 mg/kg/24h ÷q4-6h; *12-16y:* 18 mg/kg/24h ÷q6h; MAX 900 mg/24h. Serum level 10-20 mg/L

<u>zafirlukast</u> [Accolate] (Tab 20mg) >12y: 1 Tab PO BID, 1h before or 2 h after meals. **(Leukotriene receptor antagonist)**★

<u>zileuton</u> [Zyflo] (Tab 600mg) ≥12yoa: 600mg QID. **(5-lipoxygenase inhibitor inhibitor)**★

Pediatric Notes:

ANTIDEPRESSANTS (MAOI- monoamine oxidase inhibitor, SUI- serotonin uptake inhibition, TCA- tricyclic, Tetra- tetracyclic, Bul- bulemia, GAD- general anxiety disorder, OCD- obsessive-compulsive disorder)

amitriptyline [Elavil, Endep] TCA (Tab 10, 25, 50, 75, 100, 150 mg; vial 10 mg/ml) PO initially 25 mg TID or 75 mg qHS; IM 20-30 mg QID. MAX 300 mg/d

amoxapine [Asendin] TCA (Tab 25, 50, 100, 150 mg) PO 50-100 mg BID/TID, MAX 400 mg/d

bupropion [Wellbutrin] (Tab 75, 100 mg) PO initially 100 mg BID, then may increase to TID after 3 days

citalopram HBr [Celexa] SSRI (Tab 20, 40 mg) PO initial 20 mg Q D, maintenance 20-40 mg/d

clomipramine [Anafranil] TCA (Tab 25, 50, 75 mg) PO 25-100 mg QID, MAX 250 mg/d

desipramine [Norpramin] TCA (Tab 10, 25, 50, 75, 100, 150 mg) PO 25-200 mg qHS, MAX 300 mg/d

doxepin [Sinequan] TCA (Liq 10 mg/ml Tab 10, 25, 50, 75, 100, 150 mg) PO 75-150 mg qHS or BID

fluoxetine [Prozac] SUI (Tab 10 mg; Puvules 10, 20 mg★; Sol 20 mg/5ml) 20 mg QD, may use 20-40 mg BID, MAX 80 mg/d; OCD

fluvoxamine maleate [Luvox] SUI (Tab 50, 100 mg) OCD 50 mg qHS, may ↑ to 100-300 mg/d divided BID, MAX 300 mg/d

imipramine [Tofranil] (Tab 10, 25, 50 mg) PO 50-150 mg qHS, MAX 200 mg/d

isocarboxazid [Marplan] MAOI (Tab 10 mg) PO initial 10 mg BID. If tolerated, increase dosage by 10 mg every 2 to 4 days to achieve a dosage of 40 mg by the end of the first week of treatment. Increase dosage by increments of up to 20 mg/wk, if needed and tolerated, to a max of 60 mg/d. Divide into 2-4 doses/D

Limbitrol C4 [chlordiazepoxide/amitriptyline] Benzo/TCA(Tab 5/12.5, 10/25 mg) PO 1 tab TID/QID

maprotiline [Ludiomil] Tetra (Tab 25, 50, 75 mg) PO 75 mg qHS, MAX 225 mg/d

mirtazapine [Remeron] (Tab 15, 30 mg) 5 HT-1A agonist for depression,15 mg QD, titrate 15-45 mg/d

nefazodone [Serzone] SUI (Tab 100, 150, 200, 250 mg) PO 200 mg/d divided BID, maintenance 300-600 mg/d

nortriptyline [Aventyl, Pamelor] TCA (Cap 10, 25, 50, 75 mg) PO 25 mg TID/QID, MAX 100 mg/d

paroxetine [Paxil] SUI (Tab 10, 20, 30, 40 mg) *Depression:* initial 20 mg QD, may increase weekly to 50 mg QD if needed. *OCD:* initial 20 mg QD, increase weekly to 40-60 mg QD. *Panic Disorder:* initial 10 mg QD, increase weekly to 10-60 mg QD if needed. new indication for *social anxiety disorder* ★

phenelzine [Nardil] MAOI (Tab 15 mg) PO initially 15 mg TID, may increase to 90 mg/d, may reduce to 15 mg/d

protriptyline [Vivactil] TCA (Tab 5, 10 mg) PO 5-10 mg TID/QID, MAX 60 mg/d

sertraline [Zoloft] SUI (Tab 25, 50, 100 mg) PO 50-200 mg QD, MAX 200 mg/d; Bul, GAD, OCD

tranylcypromine [Parnate] MAOI (Tab 10 mg) PO 30 mg/d in divided doses, MAX 60 mg/d

trazodone [Desyrel] SUI (Tab 50, 100, 150, 300 mg) PO 50-100 mg TID, MAX 600 mg/d

trimipramine [Surmontil] TCA (Cap 25, 50, 100 mg) PO 25 mg TID, MAX 200 mg/d

venlafaxine [Effexor, Effexor XR] SUI (Tab 25, 37.5, 50, 75, 100 mg; XR 37.5, 75, 150 mg) PO 75 mg/d divided BID/TID, MAX 375 mg/d; XR Start 37.5-75 mg qd; single daily dose with food

ANTIPSYCHOTICS "Neuroleptics" (TPC- therapeutic plasma concentration. The risk of Tardive dyskinesia & irreversible effects increase as the duration of therapy and the total cumulative dose of drug increases.)

chlorpromazine [Thorazine] (Syp 10 mg/5ml; Tab 10, 25, 50, 100, 200 mg; Sup 25, 100 mg) PO/IM/PR 10-50 mg BID/TID/QID/QID; TPC 30-500 ng/ml

chlorprothixene [Taractan] (Liq 100 mg/5ml; Tab 10, 25, 50 100 mg) PO/IM 25-50 mg TID/QID

clozapine [Clozaril] (Tab 25, 100 mg) PO 25-50 mg QD, SE: agranulocytosis

etrafon [perphenazine/amitriptyline] (Tab 2/10, 2/25, 4/10, 4/25, 4mg/50 mg) PO 1 TID/QID, MAX 8 tabs/d

fluphenazine [Prolixin] (Elx 2.5 mg/5ml; Tab 1, 2.5, 5, 10 mg) PO 0.5-10 mg/d divided q6-8h; decanoate IM 12.5-25 mg q4-2 wk; TPC 0.13-2.8 ng/ml

haloperidol [Haldol](Liq 2mg/ml;Tab 0.5,1,2,5,10,20mg)PO 0.5-5mg TID;IM 2-5mg q4-8h prn; TPC 5-20 ng/ml

loxapine [Loxitane] (Cap 5, 10, 25, 50 mg) PO 10-25 mg BID; IM 12.5-50 mg q4-6h

mesoridazine [Serentil] (Liq 25 mg/ml; Tab 25, 50, 100 mg) PO 25-100 mg TID

molindone [Moban] (Liq 20 mg/ml; Tab 5, 10, 25, 50, 100 mg) PO 5-25 mg TID/QID

olanzapine [Zyprexa] (Tab 5, 7.5, 10 mg) Start with 5-10 mg PO QD, may adjust weekly by 5 mg PO QD for efficacy to 15-20 mg daily

perphenazine [Trilafon] (Liq 16 mg/5ml; Tab 2, 4, 8, 16 mg) PO 4-8 mg TID; IM 5 mg q6h; TPC 0.8-1.2 ng/ml

pimozide [Orap] (Tab 2 mg) PO 1-2 mg QD in divided doses; MAX 10 mg/d, monitor for ECG changes

quetiapine [Seroquel] (Tab 25, 100, 200 mg) *Adults >18yoa* initially 25 mg BID, increase by 25-50 mg BID or TID on days 2 & 3, by day 4 dose should be 300-400 mg/d divided BID or TID, may further increase by 25-50 mg BID or TID every 2 days to therapeutic dose. MAX 800 mg/d

risperidone [Risperdal] (Tab 1, 2, 3, 4 mg) PO day 1- 1 mg QD; day 2- 2 mg BID; day 3- 3 mg BID; then ↑ q week as needed for effect; MAX 16 mg/d

thioridazine [Mellaril] (Susp 25,100 mg/5ml; Tab 10, 15, 25, 50, 100, 150, 200 mg) PO 50-200 mg TID; MAX 800 mg/d

thiothixene [Navane] (Liq 5 mg/5ml; Tab 1, 2, 5, 10, 20 mg) PO 2-5 mg TID; IM 4 mg q6-12h; TPC 2-57 ng/ml

Triavil [perphenazine (mg)/amitriptyline (mg)] (Tab 2/10, 2/25, 4/10, 4/25, 4/50) PO 1 tab TID/QID; MAX 4 tabs of 4/50 mg/d or 8 tabs of 2/10, 2/25, 4/10, 4/25 daily

trifluoperazine [Stelazine] (Liq 10 mg/ml; Tab 1, 2, 5, 10 mg) PO 2-5 mg BID; IM 1-2 mg q4-6h

ANXIOLYTICS

<u>buspirone</u> [BuSpar] (Tab 5, 10 mg) PO 5-10 mg TID, MAX 60 mg/d

<u>hydroxyzine</u> [Atarax, Vistaril] (Tab 10, 25, 50, 100 mg; Susp 10, 25 mg/5ml) PO/IM 25-50 mg q4-6h

<u>meprobamate</u> [Equanil, Miltown, {Meprospan}] (Tab 200, 400, 600 mg; {SR 200, 400 mg}) PO 400 mg TID/QID MAX 2.4g/d; SR 400-800 mg in the morning and PM

<u>propiomazine</u> [Largon] *preop apprehension* IV/IM 20 mg with 50 mg meperidine

BENZODIAZEPINES

<u>alprazolam</u> C4 [Xanax] (Tab 0.25, 0.5, 1, 2 mg) PO 0.25-0.5 mg TID; t½ 12-15h

<u>chlordiazepoxide</u> C4 [Librium] (Tab 5, 10, 25 mg) PO 5-25 mg TID/QID; *ETOH withdrawal* IM/IV 25-100 mg q2-4h; t½ 5-30h

<u>clorazepate</u> C4 [Tranxene, Tranxene-SD] (Cap 3.75, 7.5, 15mg; Tab 3.75, 7.5, 15mg; SD 11.25, 22.5 mg) PO 7.5-15 mg qHS/BID; or maintenance 11.25-22.5 mg QD; t½ 30-100h

<u>Diastat</u> [diazepam rectal gel] (2.5, 5, 10, 15, 20 mg/applicator) Age 2-5 yrs 0.5 mg/kg/dose; 6-11yrs 0.3 mg/kg/dose; ≥12yrs 0.2 mg/kg/dose; May repeat dose in 4-12hrs.

<u>diazepam</u> C4 [Valium] (Liq 5 mg/5ml; Tab 2, 5, 10 mg) PO 2-10 mg TID/QID; IV 2.5-5 mg up to 0.2 mg/kg q3-4h prn; t½ 20-80h

<u>estazolam</u> C4 [ProSom] (Tab 1, 2 mg) PO 1-2 mg qHS

<u>flumazenil</u> [Romazicon] *Benzodiazepine overdose* IV 0.2 mg over 30sec then 0.3-0.5 mg q30sec prn; MAX 3 mg; *reverse benzodiazepine sedation* IV 0.2 mg over 15sec, then 0.2 mg qmin prn; MAX 1 mg

<u>flurazepam</u> C4 [Dalmane] (Tab 15, 30 mg) PO 15-30 mg qHS; t½ 70-90h

<u>halazepam</u> C4 [Paxipam] (Tab 20, 40 mg) PO 20-40 mg TID/QID; t½ 14h

<u>lorazepam</u> C4 [Ativan] (Tab 0.5, 1, 2 mg) PO/IM/IV 0.5-2 mg q6-8h; t½ 10-20h

<u>midazolam</u> C4 [Versed] IM 0.07 mg/kg, IV 1 mg q2-3min up to 0.1-0.15 mg/kg; *Pediatric dose for sedation, anxiolysis, or amnesia:* 0.1-0.15 mg/kg IM, may use up to 0.5 mg/kg not to exceed 10 mg; t½ 2.5h;

<u>oxazepam</u> C4 [Serax] (Tab 15; Cap 10, 15, 30 mg) PO 10-15 mg TID/QID; t½ 5-20h

<u>prazepam</u> C4 [Centrax] (Cap 5, 10, 20 mg) PO 10-20 mg TID; t½ 30-100h

<u>quazepam</u> C4 [Doral] (Tab 7.5, 15 mg) PO 1-2 tabs qHS

<u>temazepam</u> C4 [Restoril] (Tab 7.5, 15, 30 mg) PO 15-30 mg qHS; t½ 8-25h

<u>triazolam</u> C4 [Halcion] (Tab 0.125, 0.25 mg) PO 0.125-0.5 mg qHS; t½ 2-3h

other SEDATIVES, HYPNOTICS

<u>butabarbital</u> C3 [Butisol] (Elx 30 mg/5ml; Tab 15, 30, 50, 100 mg) 15-30 mg TID/QID; *insomnia* 50-100 mg HS

<u>chloral hydrate</u> C4 [Noctec] (Syp 250, 500 mg/5ml; Supp 324, 500, 648; Cap 250, 500 mg) PO 500-1000 mg *30min before HS or surgery, Sedation-* PO 250 mg TID after meals

<u>ethchlorvynol</u> C4 [Placidyl] (Tab 200, 500, 750 mg) PO 500 mg qHS, maximum duration 1 week

<u>mephobarbital</u> C4 [Mebaral] (Tab 32, 50, 100 mg) PO 32-100 mg TID/QID

<u>paraldehyde</u> [Paral] PO 4-8 ml in milk or juice

<u>pentobarbital</u> C2 [Nembutal] (Tab 50, 100 mg; Supp 30, 60, 120, 200 mg) PO 20 mg TID/QID or 100 mg HS; PR 120-200 mg; IM 150-200 mg

<u>phenobarbital</u> C4 [Solfoton] (Tab 16, 30, 100; Cap 16 mg; Elx 15, 20 mg/ml) PO 30-120 mg/d divided BID/TID

<u>zaleplon</u> C4 [Sonata] (Tab 5, 10 mg) PO 5-10 mg qHS; Elderly 5 mg qHS; MAX 20 mg★

<u>zolpidem tartrate</u> C4 [Ambien] (Tab 5, 10 mg) PO 5-10 mg qHS; MAX 10 mg

MISCELLANEOUS AGENTS

<u>Adderall</u> C2 [amphetamine/dextroamphetamine] (Tab 5, 10, 20, 30 mg) ADHD 3-5 yrs 2.5 mg daily; increase in increments of 2.5 mg/d at weekly intervals until optimal response is achieved. Usual range 0.1 to 0.5 mg/kg/dose qAM. >6 yrs - 5 mg PO qD or BID, increase in increments of 5 mg/d at weekly intervals until optimal response is achieved. Dosage rarely exceeds 40 mg/day. Usual range is 0.1 to 0.5 mg/kg/dose qAM. Give first dose on awakening; additional doses (1 or 2) may be given at 4-6h intervals.See package insert ★

<u>Biphetamine</u> C2 [amphetamine/dextroamphetamine] (Tab 6.25/6.25 mg) ADHD See insert and Adderall instructions. Long-acting forms may be used for once-a-day dosage.

<u>dextroamphetamine</u> C2 [Dexedrine] (Elx 5 mg/5ml Tab 5 mg)PO *adult narcolepsy* 5-60 mg/d in divided doses; *children ADHD 3-5yr* 2.5 mg QD; >6yr 5 mg QD, increase weekly as needed

<u>lithium carbonate</u> [Eskalith, Lithane] (Syp 300 mg/5ml; Tab 150, 300, 600 mg) PO 300 mg TID; TPC 0.6-1.2 mEq/L

<u>methamphetamine</u> C2 [Desoxyn] (Tab 5, 10, 15 mg) *ADHD children >6yr* PO initial 5 mg QD/BID, increase weekly as needed, usual dose 20-25 mg QD

<u>methylphenidate</u> C2 [Ritalin, Ritalin-SR] (Tab 5, 10, 20 mg; SR 20 mg) PO *Narcolepsy* 5-20 mg BID/TID; *ADHD children >6yr* PO initial 5 mg BID before breakfast & lunch, increase weekly as needed; MAX 60 mg QD; The Ritalin-SR has a duration of ≈8 h and may be used in place of regular tablets, SR tablets must be swallowed whole, never crushed or chewed

<u>modafinil</u> [Provigil] (Tab 100, 200 mg) 200 mg QD as single morning dose. *Narcolepsy* ★

<u>pemoline</u> C4 [Cylert] (Tab 18.75, 37.5, 75 mg) PO *ADHD children >6yr* PO initial 37.5 mg Q AM, increase weekly by 18.75 mg as needed; Max 112.5 mg QD

Asthma Classification of Severity			
Classification	Symptoms	Lung Function	Nocturnal Symptoms
Mild Intermittent	≤ 2 times a week, normal PEF and asymptomatic between brief exacerbations	FEV1 or PEF ≥ 80% predicted PEF variability < 20%	≤ twice a month
Mild Persistent	Symptoms > twice a week but < daily. Exacerbations may affect activity	FEV1 or PEF ≥ 80% predicted. PEF variability < 20-30%	> twice a month
Moderate Persistent	Daily symptoms, daily use of inhaled short-acting β₂-agonist. Exacerbations ≥ twice a week and may last for days and affects activity	FEV1 or PEF > 60 ≤ 80% predicted PEF variability < 30%	> once a week
Severe Persistent	Continual symptoms with frequent exacerbations. Limited physical activity	FEV1 or PEF ≤ 60% predicted PEF variability > 20%	Frequent
Patients should be placed in the most severe class that any of their symptoms appear. Patients frequently change severity classifications as their symptoms change.			
*Guidelines for the Diagnosis and Management of Asthma; NIH Pub 97-4051A May 97			

TRIAD ASTHMA: Severe persistent asthma, nasal polyps, aspirin or NSAID sensitivity.

PULMONARY MEDICATIONS
Key to mechanism of action and recommended use: (Li- leukotriene inhibitor, LRA- leukotriene receptor antagonist)

Anti-inflammatory (A)

Bronchodilator (B)

Reduce systemic steroid use (r)

Exercise induced asthma / environmental allergen exposure- pretreatment (e)

Acute relief / rescue for exacerbation (a)

Term- long term control and prevention of flares (t)

Hs- nocturnal symptom prevention (h)

acetylcysteine [Mucomyst] (Sol 10, 20%) HHN for mucolysis 1-10ml of 20% or 2-20ml of 10% q 2-6h
albuterol inh [Proventil, Ventolin] (Volmax ER Tab 4, 8mg; HHN 0.5%; MDI 200 dose) MDI 2 puffs q 4-6h, HHN 2.5 mg (0.5ml) (B,a,e)
albuterol oral [Elx 2mg/5ml; Tab 2, 4; Repetabs 4 mg; Volmax ER Tab 4, 8mg) PO 2-6yo 0.1mg/kg up to 2 mg TID MAX 24mg/D, adult 2-4 mg TID/QID MAX 32mg/D, Repetabs 4-8mg q 12h MAX 32mg/D, Volmax 4-8 mg q 12h (B,r,t,h)
atropine sulfate [Dey-Dose Atropine Sulfate] (Sol 0.2, 0.5%) HHN 0.025mg/kg in 3-5ml NS TID/QID, MAX 2.5mg (B,a,r,t,h)
aminophylline [Somophyllin] (Tab 100, 200, SR 225mg Liq 105mg/5ml Supp 250, 500) IV Loading Dose: 6 mg/kg over 20 min. Maintenance Dose:(Continuous IV drip) 0.5-0.7 mg/kg/hr (1gm in D₅W 250ml); Peds-see Pediatric Meds. serum level- 5-15 mcg/ml (B,t,h)
beclomethasone [Beclovent, Vanceril, Vanceril DS] (MDI 42, DS 84 μg/actuation) 2 puffs TID/QID, MAX 20 inhalations/D; Vanceril DS 2 puffs BID, MAX 10 inhalations/D (A,r,t,h)
bitolterol mesylate [Tornalate] (MDI) 2 puffs q 8h prn (B,a,e)
budesonide [Pulmicort Turbuhaler] (powder 200 mcg/actuation,) INH children >6 yo 1-2 puffs BID; adults 1-4 puffs BID. Max 800 mcg BID (inhaled steroid) (A,r,t,h)
Combivent [ipratropium bromide 18mcg + albuterol 90mcg/puff] 2 puffs QID
cromolyn sodium [Intal] (Tab 100mg,MDI 800mcg/inh)PO 200mg QID 30min before meals & HS,2 inh QID (A,e,t)
dexamethasone sodium phosphate [Decadron Phosphate Respihaler] (MDI 84mcg) 3 inh TID/QID. MAX 12 inhalations/D (A,r,t,h)
dyphylline [dihydroxypropyl theo.] (Tab 200,400; Elx 100,160mg/ml)PO≤15mg/kg q6h;IM 250-500mg q6h (B,t,h)
ephedrine sulfate (Cap 25, 50mg Inj 25, 50mg/ml) PO 25-50 mg BID/TID; IV/SC/IM 25-50mg (B,a)
epinephrine SC [Ana-Kit, Epipen] (Sol 1:1,000) SC/IM 0.01 mg/kg up to 0.3-.5 mg (0.3-0.5ml) q 20min-4h (B,a)
epinephrine, racemic [Vaponefrin] HHN 8-15 drp (B,a)
epinephrine SR [Sus-Phrine] (Sol 1:200) SC 0.1-0.3ml or children 0.005 ml/kg up to 0.15ml q 6h (B,a)
epoprostenol [Flolan] (Sol 0.5, 1.5mg) *pulmonary hypertension*; continuous chronic infusion- initial 4ng/kg/min.
ethylnorepinephrine [Bronkephrine] (2mg/ml) SC/IM 0.5-1 ml (B,a)
flunisolide [AeroBid] (MDI 250 mcg/actuation) 2 puffs BID, MAX 8 inhalations/D (A,r,t,h)

fluticasone propionate [Flovent] (MDI 44mcg/inh 7.9, 13 g; Rotadisk 50mcg/inh) Rotadisk 4-11yr 1 inh bid, max 2 inh bid; MDI >11yr 2 inh bid, Max 10 inh bid **(A,r,t,h) ★**

ipratropium [Atrovent] (MDI 18 mcg/actuation, inh sol 0.02%) inh 2 puffs QID, MAX 12 inhalations/D; Sol 2.5 ml in HHN q6h**(B,a)**

isoetharine [Bronkosol] (Sol 1%, MDI) MDI 1-2 puffs q 4h, HHN 0.25-0.5 ml of 1% in 2 ml NS q 1-4h

isoproterenol [Isuprel] (Tab 10, 15mg MDI, Sol 0.25, 0.5, 1%, 0.2mg/ml) SL 10 mg MAX 60mg/D; HHN 0.5% 5-15 inhalations; MDI 1-2 q 4-6h, IVP 0.01-0.02mg **(B,e,a)**

metaproterenol [Alupent] (Tab 10, 20mg Syp 10mg/5ml, MDI, Sol 0.4, 0.6, 5%) PO 20 mg TID/QID, MDI 2-3 puffs q 3-4h, HHN 0.01 mg/kg 5% sol up to 0.3 ml q 4h **(B,e,a)**

methylprednisolone [Medrol] (Tab 2, 4, 8, 16, 24, 32 mg) Severe persistent asthma, long-term use: PO 7.5-60 mg q d or qod(Peds 0.25-2 mg/kg/d); Asthma exacerbation (outpatient "Burst"): PEDS: 1 mg/kg q6h for 48h then 1-2mg/kg/d(max 60mg/day) in 2 divided doses until PEF ≥70% personal best or predicted;Adults-120-180 mg/d in 3-4 divided doses for 48h then 60-80 mg/d until PEF ≥ 70% personal best / predicted (3-10 days) **(A,t)**

methylprednisolone sodium succinate [Solu-Medrol] IM/IV 10-40mg q 8h or high dose 30mg/kg IV q 4-6h **(A,t)**

montelukast [Singulair] (Tab 10 mg; Chew 5 mg) PO adults 10 mg Q evening; children 6-14 years 5 mg Q evening **(Li,A,t,h)**

nedocromil sodium [Tilade] (MDI 1.75 mg/actuation) 2 inhalations QID **(A,e,t)**

oxtriphylline [Choledyl] (Sol 50, 100mg/5ml Tab 100, 200mg {SR 400, 600mg}) PO 200 mg QID {400 mg BID

pirbuterol [Maxair, Maxair autoinhaler] (MDI) MDI 1-2 puffs q 4-6h, MAX 12 puffs/D **(B,a,e)**

prednisolone [Prelone Liq] (Liq 5mg/5ml, 15mg/5ml Tab 5mg) Severe persistent asthma, long-term use: PO 7.5-60 mg q d or qod(Peds 0.25-2 mg/kg/d); Asthma exacerbation (outpatient "Burst"): PEDS: 1 mg/kg q6h for 48h then 1-2mg/kg/d (max 60mg/day) in 2 divided doses until PEF ≥ 70% personal best/predicted; Adults- 120-180 mg/d in 3-4 divided doses for 48h then 60-80 mg/d until PEF ≥ 70% personal best / predicted (3-10 days) **(A,t)**

prednisolone sodium phosphate IM/IV 4-60 mg/d **(A,t)**

prednisone [Deltasone, Liq Pred] (Elx 5mg/5ml, 5mg/ml Tab 1, 2.5, 5, 10, 20, 50mg)Severe persistent asthma, long-term use: PO 7.5-60 mg q d or qod(Peds 0.25-2 mg/kg/d); Asthma exacerbation (outpatient "Burst"): PEDS: 1 mg/kg q6h for 48h then 1-2mg/kg/d (max 60mg/day) in 2 divided doses until PEF ≥ 70% personal best or predicted; Adults- 120-180 mg/d in 3-4 divided doses for 48h then 60-80 mg/d until PEF ≥ 70% personal best or predicted (3-10 days) **(A,t)**

salmeterol [Serevent] (MDI 25 mcg/actuation) 2 inhalations BID **(B,e,t,h)**

terbutaline [Brethine, Bricanyl] (Tab 2.5, 5mg; MDI) PO 2.5-5 mg TID MAX 15mg/D, SC 0.25 mg may repeat in 15-30 min, MAX 0.5 mg per 4 h period; MDI 2 puffs q 4-6h Use caution in patient with coronary artery disease, do not use in pediatrics. **(B,a,e)**

theophylline [Elixophyllin, Slo-Phyllin] (Liq 80mg/15ml Tab 100, 125, 200, 250, 300mg Cap 100, 200mg) Peds see Pediatric Meds; PO loading 5mg/kg, Maintenance 3mg/kg/8h. Serum level- 5-15 mcg/ml **(B,t,h)**

theophylline extended release [Uni-Dur] (Tab 400, 600 mg) PO 1QD. Serum level- 5-15 mcg/ml **(B,t,h)**

theophylline SR [Slo-bid, Theo-Dur] (Tab 50, 75, 100mg, 200, 300, 450 mg) Peds see Pediatric Meds; PO 100-300 mg BID. Serum level- 5-15 mcg/ml **(B,t,h)**

triamcinolone acetonide [Azmacort] (MDI 100 mcg/actuation) 2 puffs TID/QID, MAX 16 inhalations/D **(A,r,t,h)**

zafirlukast [Accolate] (Tab 10★, 20mg) PO 7-11 yrs 10mg BID; >11 yrs 20mg PO BID 1 hour before or 2 h after meals. **(LRA,A,t,h)**

zileuton [Zyflo] (Tab 600mg) ≥12yoa: 600mg QID. **(5-lipoxygenase inhibitor inhibitor,A,t,h)**

PNEUMONIA- COMMUNITY ACQUIRED:

PREDICTING RISKS FROM COMMUNITY-ACQUIRED PNEUMONIA (NEJM,1997; 336:243-250)

SCORING SYSTEM FOR PREDICTION MODEL

PATIENT CHARACTERISTIC	POINTS	Laboratory	
Demographics		PH <7.35	+30
Males	Age in years	BUN >10.7 mmol/L	+20
Females	Age in years - 10	Na+ <130 mEq/L	+20
Comorbid Illnesses		Glucose >13.9 mmol/L	+10
Neoplastic disease	+30	Hematocrit <30%	+10
Liver disease	+20	PO2 <60 mmHg	+10
CHF	+10	Pleural effusion	+10
Cerebrovascular disease	+10	**STRATIFICATION OF RISK SCORE**	
Physical Exam		Risk	Risk Class	Based on
Altered mental status	+20	Low	I	Algorithm
Respiratory rate ≥30/min	+20	Low	II	≤70 points
Systolic blood pressure <90mmHg	+20	Low	III	71-90 points
Temp <35°C or ≥40°C	+15	Moderate	IV	91-130 points
Pulse ≥125 bpm/min	+10	High	V	>130 points

AMERICAN THORACIC SOCIETY'S GUIDELINES for the initial management of adults with community acquired pneumonia: diagnosis, assessment of severity and initial antimicrobial therapy. *Am Resp Dis.*1993;148:1418-1426

<60 y: •DDX- Strep pneumonia, M. pneumonia, H. influenza, C. pneumonia, viral, legionella, C. psittaci
- •**R**: outpatient treatment based on most likely organisms- erythromycin 500mg qid or azithromycin 500mg day 1 then 250mg qd or clarithromycin 500 mg bid or doxycycline 100 mg bid. Treat Strep pneumonia until afebrile for 3 days, treat M. pneumonia for 2-3 wks.

>60 y: •DDX- Strep pneumonia, respiratory virus, H. influenza, aerobic gram neg bacilli; legionella
- •Findings supporting hospitalization versus outpatient treatment: >65 yr, co-existing illnesses, previous pneumonia <1 year prior, altered mental status, alcohol abuse, aspiration, splenectomy, Temp >101°F, extra-pulmonary infection, WBC <4,000>30,000, PaCO2>50, sepsis, HCT<30, pleural effusion. Finding supporting ICU admission: **possible need for intubation, multiple lobes involved, PaO2<60 or pO2 Sat <90%, reps rate >30, shock, acute renal failure**

<u>Classification</u>
Category 1: Mild-moderate (<2 risk factors), outpatient treatment, < 60y, no comorbidity
Category 2: Mild-moderate, outpatient treatment, < 60y, + comorbidity
Mild-moderate, outpatient treatment, ≥ 60y, - comorbidity
Category 3: Moderate, admit to ward, +/- comorbidity
Category 4: Severe (reps ≥30, BP<90/60, parapneumonic effusion, O2 Sat <90%) admit to ICU
- •**R**: <u>outpatient-</u> erythromycin 500mg qid or azithromycin 500mg day 1 then 250mg qd or clarithromycin 500 mg bid for 7-10 days plus ampicillin/clavulanate 875 mg PO bid or cefuroxime axetil 500 mg PO BID (or other 2nd or 3rd generation ceph) or trimethoprim/sulfamethoxazole 1 DS tab PO BID for 7-10 days
<u>hospitalized-</u> .
- •Stable- erythromycin 20mg/kg/24h IV divided q 6h or azithromycin 500mg IV qd plus or cefuroxime 750 mg-1.5g IV q8h (or other 2nd or 3rd generation ceph)
- •Severe- (resp rate >30, multiple lobes involved, PaO2<60) cefotaxime 2gm IV q8h or ceftriaxone 2gm IV qd plus erythromycin 1gm IV q6h; or meropenem IV 0.5-1gm or ticarcillin/clavulanate 3.1 gm IV q 4-6h or piperacillin/tazobactam 3.375g IVPB q 6h plus erythromycin 1gm IV q6h

Hospital Acquired: DDX- Pseudomonas, E. coli, Klebsiella, Enterobacter, Acinetobacter, legionella
- •**R** meropenem IV 0.5-1gm q8h or imipenem/cilastatin1gm IVPB q 6-8h

---

CHEST X-RAY INTERPRETATION
"ALWAYS APPROACH THE CXR IN A SYSTEMATIC MANNER"

<u>POSITION</u> The spinous processes of the vertebrae should be midline in the trachea air column. Clavicular heads should be equal distances from the spinous processes. Rotation will distort the view of the hilar complexes, mediastinum and heart configuration and may result in false interpretation of pathology.
<u>SOFT TISSUE</u> Check for subcutaneous air, symmetry, tissue planes and swelling.
<u>SKELETAL STRUCTURES</u> Examine the sternum, clavicles, scapulas, ribs and vertebrae. Look for fractures, arthritic changes, rib notching, osteolytic or osteoblastic lesions.
<u>DIAPHRAGM</u> Hemidiaphragms should be equal and rounded. A high hemidiaphragm suggests paralysis, flattening suggests COPD. Costophrenic angles should be sharp and free of fluid (>300ml present to be evident on CXR). Check below the diaphragm for free air and gas pattern. Spleen calcification suggests histoplasmosis.
<u>HEART and MEDIASTINUM</u> Check for the normal three humps: aortic knob, pulmonary conus and LV. A fourth hump suggests Left atrial enlargement. The heart should be less than half the chest width (>1/2 CHF, pericardial fluid). Mediastinal widening suggests thoracic aorta disruption, mass, or pericardial fluid. Tracheal deviation suggests tension pneumothorax, tumor, or atelectasis. **Mediastinal Mass**: Anterior- Thymus, Teratoma, Substernal Thyroid, Lymphoma; Posterior- Neurogenic tumor, Lymphoma.
<u>HILAR COMPLEXES</u> Left hilum 2-3 cm higher. Right hilum is never higher without pathology. Should be equal density (increased density suggests bronchiogenic CA). **Bilateral Hilar Adenopathy**: Sarcoid, Lymphoma, Histoplasmosis.
<u>LUNG FIELDS</u> Should be "clear" with normal lung markings to the perimeter. Vessels should get smaller in upper lung. "Silhouette sign"- obliteration of the heart border means the lesion is anterior in the chest in the RML, anterior segment of upper lobe or lingula. Posterior lesions will show a radiopacity that overlaps the heart border.
ATELECTASIS, SIGNS OF: Major: crowding of lung markings, movement of lobar fissures. Minor: consolidation, deviation of anatomical structures, elevation of the hemidiaphragm.
BOWING OF THE LOBAR FISSURES: Cancer, Lung abscess, Klebsiella pneumonia.
CAVITARY LESIONS: TB, abscess, cancer, coccidioidomycosis.
COIN LESIONS: DDX- granuloma [TB, histoplasmosis ("Target" calcified lesion), coccidioidomycosis], carcinoma, metastatic dz, hamartoma ("Popcorn" calcifications)

COPD: Hyperlucent fields, flat diaphragms, small heart. <u>Complications</u>: Bronchospasm, Hypoxia, Secretions, Infection, Cor Pulmonale.

EXTRAPLEURAL LESIONS: DDX- rib mites, lung CA, mesothelioma, pulmonary infarction.

HEART FAILURE: Larger vessels in upper lung ("cephalization"), cardiomegaly, pulmonary edema, Kerley B lines. <u>Kerley B Lines</u>- Thickening of the interlobular septa appear as linear densities found at the lateral base of the lung, due to cellular infiltration or pulmonary edema. DDX: Acute CHF, Pneumoconiosis, Mitral Valve disease, Lymphangitic Mets.

INFILTRATE

<u>Interstitial</u>: Ground glass pattern, reticular pattern, nodular densities.
Acute: Interstitial edema, viral or mycoplasma pneumonia.
Chronic Upper lobe: Fungal, TB, eosinophilic granuloma, inhalational.
Chronic Lower lobe: DDX- "BADASS"- Bronchiectasis, Aspiration, Disseminated Interstitial Pneumonia, Asbestosis, Silicosis, Scleroderma.
Chronic Diffuse: DDX- infectious, neoplasm, congenital, vascular, inhalational, immunological, idiopathic, drug induced.
"Honeycomb lung"- End stage fibrosis. DDX: Sarcoidosis, histiocytosis, rheumatoid lung, eosinophilic granuloma, other chronic fibrosis.
<u>Alveolar</u>: Butterfly pattern, fluffy margins, air bronchogram, quick progression, segmental or lobar distribution. DDX: Acute- pneumonia, edema, hemorrhage; Chronic- sarcoidosis, lymphoma, alveolar cell CA.
<u>White-out</u>: DDX- Effusion, Atelectasis, Consolidation.

KARTAGENER'S SYNDROME: Heredity, Sinusitis, bronchiectasis, situs inversus viscerum.

LYMPHANGITIC METASTASIS: DDX- Above Diaphragm: lung, breast, thyroid, larynx. Below Diaphragm: stomach, pancreas.

LYMPHOMA: Peribronchial infiltrate, Extension from hilar nodes, pulmonary nodules, Patchy or homogenous infiltrate.

METASTASIS TO THE LUNG: Thyroid, renal, uterine, lymphoma, melanoma, mycosis fungoides, ovarian CA.

PLEURAL EFFUSION: Vascular markings seen behind the effusion (subpulmonic effusion appears as a raised or thickened hemidiaphragm).

	Transudate	Exudate
LDH	< 200	> 200
LDH pleural/plasma	< 0.6	> 0.6
Total Protein g/dl	< 3.0	> 3.0
Total Protein pleural/plasma	< 0.5	> 0.5

Bloody Effusion: DDX- Lung carcinoma, Pulmonary Emboli, Trauma.

PNEUMOTHORAX: Lung markings should extend to the periphery. Always rule out pneumothorax!

PULMONARY EMBOLUS: Dyspnea, tachypnea, tachycardia, cough, hemoptysis. CXR - wedge sign. ECG- $S_1Q_3L_3$ pattern. ABG's- not reliable. Ventilation-Perfusion Scan- screen. Angiography- definitive, "Gold Standard".

RHEUMATOID LUNG CHARACTERISTICS: Pleural effusion, interstitial fibrosis, necrobiotic nodule, Kaplan's syndrome (coal miner's pneumoconiosis).

S SIGN OF GOLDEN: Pathognomonic for upper lobe cancer.

SARCOID STAGES: Stage I: Hilar adenopathy; Stage II: Peripheral infiltrate plus stage I; Stage III: Resolving hilar adenopathy and stage II; Stage IV: Diffuse interstitial fibrosis.

SILICOSIS: "Egg shell" calcification.

UPPER LOBE PATHOLOGY: Tuberculosis, pneumoconiosis, fungus.

YELLOW NAIL SYNDROME (congenital lymphatic hypoplasia): Sinusitis, bronchiectasis, yellow nails, lymphedema.

Pulmonary Notes:

ANTINUCLEAR ANTIBODY (ANA) FREQUENCY*

Disease	% frequency of Antibodies									
	ANA	DS-DNA	Histone	RNP	Ro	La	SM	Centromere	Sci-79	PM-1
SLE	95-99	20-30	70	30-50	30	15	30	<5		
Drug induced SLE	100		95	15	50	25				
Neonatal SLE (mothers)					100	10				
Sjogren's	95	<5		15	55	90				
Scleroderma	50			30	5	<5				
Diffuse				15					20-60	
CREST				10				>80		
RA	13-35		20	10	10	5				
Polymyositis	30-50			10	15					50
MCTD	95-99			95	<5	<5				

*adapted from Primer on the Rheumatic Diseases, Tenth Edition 1993 and Internal Medicine for the Specialist 1987;8:59-68

**The percentage of a population with a specific HLA type that will have the associated disease.

HLA ASSOCIATIONS*

Disease	HLA Type	% Positive	Relative Risk**
Ankylosing Spondylitis	B27	90	50
Reiter's Syndrome	B27	75	37
Sjogren's Syndrome	DR3	70	10
SLE	DR3	58	6
Scleroderma	DR5	35	5
Rheumatoid Arthritis	DR4	38	4

SYSTEMIC LUPUS ERYTHEMATOSUS CRITERIA* (≥4 Findings for diagnosis)

Criterion	Definition
Malar rash	Fixed erythema over malar eminence, tending to spare the nasolabial folds.
Discoid rash	Erythematous raised patches with keratotic scaling & follicular plugging.
Photosensitivity	Unusual skin rash due to sunlight - Pt. History of Dr. observation.
Oral ulcers	Oral or nasopharyngeal, usually painless – observed by Dr.
Arthritis	Nonerosive in ≥2 peripheral joints (+tenderness, swelling, or effusion).
Serositis	Pleuritis, OR, pericarditis
Renal disorder	Proteinuria >500 mg/24h or >3+, OR, Cellular casts
Neurologic disorder	Seizures, OR, Psychosis (both in absence of offending drugs or metabolic derangement's)
Hematologic disorder	Hemolytic anemia (with reticulocytosis), OR, Leukopenia (<4000/mm³), OR, Lymphopenia (<1500/mm³), OR, Thrombocytopenia (<100,000/mm³).
Immunologic disorder	(+) LE cell prep, OR, Anti-DNA, OR, Anti-Sm, OR, False (+) VDRL X 6 mos.
Antinuclear antibody	At any time in the absence of "drug-induced lupus."

CLASSIFICATION OF RHEUMATOID ARTHRITIS (1987 American Rheumatism Association criteria)

Criterion	Definition
a. Morning stiffness	In & around joints ≥1h before maximal improvement
b. Arthritis in ≥3 joints	Soft tissue swelling or fluid (not bony overgrowth alone) seen by a physician. 14 possible areas: R or L PIP, MCP, wrist, elbow, knee, ankle, & MTP joints.
c. Arthritis of hand joints	≥1 area swollen in wrist, MCP, or PIP.
d. Symmetric arthritis	Simultaneous joint involvement on both sides of body.
e. Rheumatoid nodules	Subcutaneous nodules over bony prominence, extensor surfaces, or Juxta-articular.
f. Serum rheumatoid factor	Abnormal amounts of RF.
g. Radiographic changes	PA hand & wrist X-rays (erosions, decalcification next to involved joints).

a-d must be present ≥6 weeks; b-e must be observed by a physician. (≥4 Findings for diagnosis)

SLOW-ACTING ANTIRHEUMATIC DRUGS (SAARD's) **See current guidelines for dosing and monitoring**

auranofin [Ridaura] (Cap 3 mg) PO 3 mg BID, OR, 6 mg QD. (usual peak response 6 mos.)

aurothioglucose [Solganal] (Inj 50 mg/ml) Weekly IM injections of: 1st dose 10 mg, 2nd & 3rd doses 25 mg, subsequent doses 50 mg. Max 1000 mg cumulative

azathioprine [Imuran] (Tab 50 mg; Inj 100 mg) Initially 1 mg/kg PO/IV daily, then increase gradually. MAX 2.5 mg/kg/day

etanercept [Enbrel] (25 mg vials) *Adults:* 25 mg given twice weekly as an SC injection. *Children (4-17 yoa):* 0.4 mg/kg SC twice weekly for 3 months (Max 25 mg). Recombinant TNF for moderate to severe RA who had inadequate response to DMARDS ★

hydroxychloroquine [Plaquenil] (Tab 200 mg) *Lupus-* Initial 400 mg q12-24h, maintenance 200-400 mg/24h; *rheumatoid arthritis-* Initial 400-600 mg/24h, maintenance 200-400 mg/24h.

leflunomide [Arava] (Tab 10, 20, 100 mg) PO 100 mg QD for 3 days, then 20 mg QD

methotrexate [Rheumatrex] (Tab 2.5 mg; Inj 25 mg/ml) 7.5 mg PO/IM/IV q wk, or 2.5 mg PO q12h X 3 q wk

penicillamine [Cuprimine, Depen] (Cap 125, 250 mg; Tab 250 mg) Initially 125-250 mg/day, then, gradually increase to a MAX 750 mg/day

salicylate [Trilisate, choline magnesium trisalicylate] (Tab 500, 750 mg; Liq 500 mg/5ml) PO 3gm HS or + BID.

sulfasalazine [Azulfidine EN-tabs] (Tab 500 mg) *Adults* 2g daily in evenly divided doses. Titrate dose over 4wk

Synvisc [hylan G-F20] treatment consists of 3 intra-articular injections given at 1 week intervals

AGENTS FOR GOUT

Col-Probenecid [Tab probenecid 500 mg + colchicine 0.5 mg) *Initial* 1 tab PO QD X 1 week, then 1 tab PO BID.

probenecid [Benemid] (Tab 0.5 g) PO 0.25 g BID X 1 week, then, 0.5 g BID.

sulfinpyrazone [Anturane] (Tab 100 mg; Cap 200 mg) PO 200-400 mg daily in 2 divided doses.

allopurinol [Zyloprim] (Tab 100, 300 mg) PO 200-600 mg/24h in divided doses.

colchicine (Tab 0.5, 0.6 mg; Inj 1 mg) *Acute flare:* 0.5-1.2 mg PO q1-2h, OR, initially 2 mg IV, then, 0.5 mg IV q6h until pain is relieved, nausea, vomiting or diarrhea occurs.

Rheumatology Notes:

TOXICOLOGY / DEPENDENCY

<u>acetylcysteine</u> [Mucomyst] *acetaminophen toxicity:* loading PO or NGT 140 mg/kg of 20% solution, then 70 mg/kg q4h x 17 doses

<u>bupropion</u> [Zyban] (Tab 150 mg) *Initially* 1 tab QD X 3days, ↑ to 1 tab BID, treat 7-12 wks. *Smoking cessation*

<u>charcoal</u> PO 30-100 grams, 1 g/kg. *Peds* 15-30 g, If it contains sorbitol, no cathartic is needed. If not, use: magnesium citrate 4cc/kg (MAX 200cc)

<u>deferoxamine mesylate</u> [Desferal] *Acute iron intoxication:* IM 1 g then 0.5 g q4h for 2 doses, Chronic overload: IM 0.5-1 g/D, IV 2 g with each unit of blood, SC 1-2 g/d over 8-24h with continuous infusion pump

<u>digoxin Immune Fab</u> [Digibind] (40 mg/vial) IV 2-20 vials, 1 vial will bind 0.6 mg of digoxin

<u>dimercaprol</u> [BAL] *arsenic or gold poisoning* 2.5 mg/kg IM QID for 2d, then BID on third day, then qd for 10d; *lead poisoning* 4 mg/kg first doses then q4h with calcium edetate disodium for 2-7d; *mercury poisoning* 5 mg/kg initially then 2.5 mg/kg qd/BID for 10d

<u>disulfiram</u> [Antabuse] (Tab 250, 500 mg) PO Initially 500 mg QD for 1-2 wks then 250-500 mg QD

<u>edetate calcium disodium</u> [EDTA] *lead toxicity* IM 35 mg/kg BID, PEDS divided daily dose q8-12h

<u>ethanol</u> *ethylene glycol & methanol toxicity:* PO or IV infusion to maintain an ethanol level of 100 mg/dl

<u>flumazenil</u> [Romazicon] *benzodiazepine overdose* IV 0.2 mg over 30sec then 0.3-0.5 mg q30sec prn, MAX 3 mg; *reverse benzodiazepine sedation* IV 0.2 mg over 15sec then 0.2 mg qmin prn, MAX 1 mg

<u>ipecac</u> PO 1-12yrs: 15ml + 300ml water; >12yrs: 30ml + 300ml water

<u>nalmefene</u> [Revex] (100 mcg/ml, 1 mg/ml)IV 0.25 mcg/KG, then q2-5min until *opioid reversal* is obtained; cumulative total dose >1 mcg/kg does not provide additional therapeutic effect; SC/IM 1 mg if IV access lost.

<u>naloxone</u> [Narcan] (0.2, 0.4 & 1.0 mg/ml) IM/IV 5-10 mcg/kg/dose q3-5 min prn. MAX 2 mg.

<u>naltrexone</u> [Revia] (Tab 50 mg) PO *Alcoholism* 50 mg QD. *Narcotic dependence-* (must be opioid free for at least 7-10 days before starting) 25 mg initial dose then 50 mg QD if no withdrawal symptoms after initial dose.

<u>nicotine gum</u> [Nicorette 2, DS 4 mg (96 pieces)] 9-12 pieces/d

<u>nicotine patches</u> [Habitrol, Nicoderm 7, 14, 21 mg/d; Nicotrol 5, 10, 15 mg/d; Prostep 11, 22 mg] Nicoderm 21 mg patch/d for 6 wks, then 14 mg/d for 2wks then 7 mg/d for 2wks

<u>Nicotine nasal spray</u> [Nicotrol NS] (metered spray 10mg/ml; 0.5 mg nicotine/spray) 1 spray each nostril 1-2 times/hr; Min recommended dose is 8 doses/d; Max recommended dose is 40 doses/d

<u>Nicotrol Nicotine inhaler</u> nicotine inhalation system- 42 cartridges each containing 10 mg (4 mg is delivered) nicotine. The initial dosage of NICOTROL Inhaler is individualized. Patients may self-titrate to the level of nicotine they require. Most successful patients use 6-16 cartridges a day. Best effect is achieved by frequent continuous puffing (20 minutes). The recommended duration of treatment is 3 months, after which patients may be weaned by gradual reduction of the daily dose over the following 6 to 12 wks

<u>penicillamine</u> [Cuprimine] (Tab 125, 250 mg) *Wilson's disease* 1 g/d on empty stomach divided QID

<u>physostigmine salicylate</u> [Antilirium] *anticholinergic toxicity* (TCA) IV/IM 2 mg

<u>pralidoxime chloride</u> [2-PAM] *Organophosphate toxicity* IV 1-2 g over 15-30 min in 100ml NS, may give IM/SC

<u>sodium thiosulfate</u> (12.5 g/50cc amp) *arsenic toxicity* initially 1 ml, then 2, 3, and 4 ml on successive days; *cyanide toxicity* slow IVP 12.5g over 10min after sodium nitrate IV 300 mg

Toxicology Notes:

UROLOGY

alprostadil [Caverject, Edex] (Inj 5, 10, 20, 40mcg/vial) *Vasculogenic, psychogenic, or mixed* Initial 2.5 mcg over 5-10 seconds into the lateral aspect of proximal 3rd of penis. *Neurogenic* Initial 1.25 mcg. Titrate in the physician's office for erection sufficient for intercourse and <1h duration. Max 40 mcg and 3 self-injections/week. Allow at least 24° between doses.

ammonium chloride (Tab 500 mg) PO 1 gm TID up to 6 days, acidifier

bethanechol chloride [Urecholine] (Tab 5, 10, 25, 50 mg) PO 10-50 mg TID/QID, SC 5 mg TID/QID, cholinergic

desmopressin [DDAVP] (5ml Nasal pump 10 mcg/spray; Inj 4 mcg/ml) nocturnal enuresis (>6yoa) initial 10mcg each nostril qHS, then adjust to effect up to 40 mcg daily; 4-8 weeks

Detrol [tolterodine](Tab 1, 2 mg) PO initial 2 mg BID; maybe lowered to 1 mg BID

dimethyl sulfoxide [DMSO] (Sol 50%) 50 ml instilled into bladder for 15 min q2wks

finasteride [Proscar] (Tab 5 mg) PO 5 mg QD

flavoxate [Urispas] (Tab 100 mg) PO 100-200 mg TID/QID, antispasmodic

neostigmine methylsulfate [Prostigmin] (Sol 0.25, 0.5, 1 mg/ml) SC/IM 0.5 mg for retention, may repeat after catheter placement 0.5 mg q5h for at least 5 injections.

Nilandron [nilutamide] (Tab 50 mg) PO 6 tabs QD 30 days followed thereafter by 3 tabs QD; can be taken with or without food; indicated for use in combination with surgical castration for the treatment of metastatic prostate cancer (Stage D2)

oxybutynin chloride [Ditropan] (Tab 5 mg; Syp 5 mg/5ml) Adults PO 5 mg BID/TID, MAX 5 mg QID; Pediatric patients over 5yoa PO 5 mg BID, MAX 5 mg TID, antispasmodic, anticholinergic

pentosan polysulfate sodium [Elmiron] (Cap 100 mg) 100 mg PO TID. TX bladder pain from interstitial cystitis

phenazopyridine [Pyridium] (Tab 100, 200 mg) PO 200 mg TID (2 days)

potassium acid phosphate [K-Phos] (Tab 500 mg) PO 1gm in 180 ml water with meals & HS, Acidifier

potassium citrate [Urocit-K] (Tab 5 mEq) PO 10-20 mEq TID with meals, alkalinizer

sodium bicarbonate (Tab 325, 650 mg) PO 325-2,000 mg up to QID, MAX 17 mg/D, alkalinizer

tamsulosin [Flomax] (Cap 0.4 mg) 0.4 mg ½hr after same meal QD, ↑ to 0.8 mg after 2-4wks if needed.

Viagra [sildenafil] (Tab 25, 50, 100 mg) PO initial dose 50 mg 1 hour before sexual activity, Max 100 mg qd

yohimbine HCl [Yocon] (Tab 5.4 mg) PO 1 tab TID

Zoladex [goserelin acetate/futamide] (10.8 mg) management of locally confined stage B2-C prostate carcinoma in combination with flutamide

Urology Notes:

VACCINES / IMMUNOGLOBULINS

antivenin (crotalidae) polyvalent Rattlesnake. Perform sensitivity test first. Minimal envenomation: IV 20-40 ml (2-4 vials); Moderate: 50-90 ml; Severe: 100-150 ml. IM may be used only if IV access cannot be obtained.

antivenin (micrurus fulvius) polyvalent North American Coral Snake. IV drip 250-500ml NS, 30-50 ml of antivenin by slow IV push, inject first 1-2 ml over 3-5 min, if no signs of reaction then complete the injection.

basiliximab [Simulect] IV BID; IL-2 receptor antagonist for organ rejection in renal transplant

cholera vaccine endemic or epidemic areas: SC/IM 2 doses 1wk apart, *6m-4y* 0.2 ml, *5-10y* 0.3 ml, *>10y* 0.5 ml

cytomegalovirus immune globulin, human [CMV-IGIV] associated with kidney transplant IV 150mg/kg if within 72h of transplant, 2-8 wks after transplant 100 mg/kg, 12-16 wks 50 mg/kg, start at 15 mg/kg/hr then up to 60 mg/kg/hours

daclizumab [Zenapax] 5 times a day; IL-2 receptor antagonist for organ rejection in renal transplant

diptheria antitoxin treatment of Diptheria: IM/slow IV 20,000-120,000U depending on severity and length of time since onset; Prophylaxis: for all unimmunized contacts IM 10,000U then immunize with diptheria toxoid. Perform sensitivity tests before administering antitoxin.

diptheria-tetanus toxoid Pediatrics <6y: DT 0.5 ml doses, see Pediatrics for schedule; *Adults, >7y*: (Td) primary-two doses of 0.5 ml 4-8 wks apart, then a third dose 6-12 mos later. Wound management see ER section

diptheria-tetanus toxoid & pertussis vaccine (whole cell) [DTP] Primary immunization 6 wk to 6 yo: IM 0.5 ml on three occasions, starting at 6 weeks of age, then a 4-8 week intervals with a reinforcing dose 1 yr after the third injection. Booster: IM 0.5ml at 4-6yr of age. Future boosters-use diphtheria and tetanus toxoid every 10yr

hemophilus B vaccine IM HibTITER 2-6m three 0.5ml inj ≈2m apart; PedvaxHIB 2-14m two 0.5ml inj ≈2m apart; ProHIBit 15m-5y single 0.5ml injection

hepatitis A Vaccine [Havrix] (720 EL.U/0.5ml, 1440 EL.U/ml) Adults deltoid IM 1440 EL.U.; *Peds 2-18yoa* 720 EL.U. Booster- repeat dose is recommended after 6-18 months to ensure highest titers

hepatitis A vaccine [Vaqta] (vials/syringes 25 U/0.5ml, 50 U/1ml) Deltoid IM. Adults 1cc; *Peds (ages 2-17yoa)* 0.5cc. Booster- repeat dose is recommended after 6-18 months to ensure highest titers

hepatitis B immune globulin [H-BIG, Nabi-HB★] post exposure prophylaxis IM 0.06 ml/kg, repeat in 28-30 days

hepatitis B Vaccine [Recombivax HB, {Engerix-B}] deltoid IM, Birth-10yoa 2.5mcg {10mcg} doses, 11-19 yoa 5mcg {20mcg} doses,>20yoa 10mcg {20mcg}doses; at 0, 1, 6 months

immune globulin, IGIV [Sandoglobulin] Immunodeficiency IV 200 mg/kg q month

influenza vaccine [Fluzone, Flushield, Fluvirin] September or October for high risk patients: IM >12yoa 0.5 ml

Lyme Disease Vaccine [LYMErix] (30 mcg/0.5 ml recombinant lipoprotein OspA on aluminum hydroxide adjuvant; single-dose vials and prefilled syringes) ★

meningococcal polysaccharide vaccine [Menomune-A/C/Y/W-135] >2yoa at risk in epidemic or highly endemic areas; consider in household contacts, medical personnel at risk of exposure, travel to epidemic area, terminal complement component deficiency patients, asplenia patients. SC 0.5 ml

measles, mumps & rubella vaccine [MMR] SC 0.5 ml, see the following immunization schedule

palivizumab [Synagis] monoclonal antibody for the prevention of serious lower respiratory tract disease in pediatric patients at high risk of RSV disease

Pneumococcal vaccine [Pneumovax] SC/IM 0.5 ml. Recommended for the following groups:

"A" *recommendations* (strong epidemiologic evidence and substantial clinical benefit supports vaccine use)
- persons ≥ 65 years of age. Revaccination if initial dose was > 5 years previously and was < 65 years old at 1st dose.
- immunocompetent persons 2-64 years of age who are at increased risk due to chronic illness (diabetes, chronic cardiovascular disease, chronic pulmonary disease). Revaccination not recommended.
- persons 2-64 years of age with functional or anatomic asplenia. If patient is > 10 years old - single revaccination if ≥ 5 years after initial dose. If patient is ≤ 10 years old, consider revaccination 3 years after initial dose.

"B" *recommendation* (moderate evidence supports vaccine use)
- persons 2-64 years of age with alcoholism, chronic liver disease or CSF leaks. Revaccination is not recommended

"C" *recommendation* (effectiveness is not proven, but the potential benefits justify vaccination)
- persons 2-64 years of age living in environments in which the risk for disease is high (including certain American Indian populations and Alaskan natives). Revaccination not recommended.
- immunocompromised persons ≥ 2years of age†. Single revaccination if ≥ 5 years since initial dose. If patient is ≤ 10 years old, consider revaccination 3 years after initial dose.

† including- HIV, lymphoma, leukemia, multiple myeloma, malignancy, Hodgkin's disease, chronic renal failure, Nephrotic syndrome, organ transplant recipients receiving immunosuppressive chemotherapy.

MMWR, 46:1-24, 1997 APR 4

polio vaccine, oral [Orimune] Primary three 0.5 ml doses, see following schedule

rabies immune globulin [Imogam] Postexposure: IM 20 IU/kg, up to the 8th day after 1st dose of vaccine

rabies vaccine, HDCV [Imovax] Postexposure: IM five 1ml doses on day 0, 3, 7, 14, 28; along with RIG on day 0 respiratory syncytial virus immune globulin intravenous [RSV-IGIV] human (Inj 2500mg) IV infusion, max dose 750mg/kg- 1.5ml/kg/hr for 15 min, then 3ml/kg/hr for 15 min, then 6ml/kg/hr

rotavirus [Rotashield] (oral susp) live, oral, tetravalent vaccine for prevention of gastroenteritis due to rotavirus. Should be offered to all healthy full-term infants, unless contraindicated★ 7/15/99 the CDC recommended *that healthcare providers and parents postpone use of the rotavirus vaccine for infants, at least until November 1999, based on early surveillance reports of intussusception ★

rubella vaccine see current recommendation

RHO immune globulin [RhoGAM] Antepartum IM 300 mcg at 26-28 wks and repeat within 72h after Rh-incompatible delivery; Postpartum prophylaxis IM 300 mcg within 72h after delivery

tetanus antitoxin treatment of tetanus: IV/IM 50,000-100,000u, give at least part of the dose IV; prevention when TIG is not available: IM/SC <29.5kg 1500, >29.5kg 3000-5000u, protection lasts <15 days.

tetanus immune globulin [Hyper-Tet] IM *Adults* 250 u, *Children* 4u/kg or may use adult dose

tetanus toxoid Primary immunization: IM two 0.5 ml doses 4-8 wks apart

tuberculin PPD [Tubersol] intradermal (Mantoux test) 5 tuberculin units; read at 48-72h, induration ≥10mm is positive, 5-9mm is inconclusive- retest at a different site; in a patient with known contacts 5mm is positive.

typhoid vaccine >6yoa: expected intimate exposure to person with typhoid, travels to high risk area, lab worker with contact: PO primary 1 capsule on days 1, 3, 5, 7 with water, one h before meal.

varicella-zoster immune globulin [VZIG] post varicella exposure IM 125u/10kg, Min 125u, MAX 635u

varicella vaccine [Varivax] chickenpox: 0.5ml SC, *age ≥13yrs* add 0.5ml booster 4-8 wks after initial inj.

yellow fever vaccine [YF Vax] immunity begins on 10th day, repeat q 10y if needed: SC 0.5 ml

PEDIATRIC IMMUNIZATION SCHEDULE- Clinical Reviews 8(9):128-130, 1998.

Vaccine	AGE IN MONTHS								YEARS		
	Birth	1	2	4	6	12	15	18	4-6	11-12	14-16
Hepatitis B	Hep B-1										
		Hep B-2			Hep B-3				★		
DTP			DTaP[1]	DTaP	DTaP		DTaP		DTaP	Td	
H influenza b			Hib	Hib	Hib	Hib					
Poliovirus			Polio[2]	Polio		Polio			Polio		
MMR						MMR			MMR	★	
Varicella						Varicella				★	

Shaded area indicates acceptable age ranges.

[1]Diphtheria and tetanus toxoids and acellular pertussis (DTaP) vaccine is preferred vaccine for all doses. Diphtheria and tetanus toxoids and whole-cell pertussis vaccine, adsorbed (DTP) may be used.

[2]Three options: 1) Two doses of Inactivated Polio Virus vaccine (IPV) followed by two doses of Oral Polio Virus (OPV); 2) four doses of IPV; 3) four doses of OPV

★Administer Varicella vaccine to 11-12 year olds not previously vaccinated and who lack a reliable history of chicken pox. Administer Hepatitis B vaccine series to 11-12 year olds not previously vaccinated. Administer 2nd MMR if not previously given.

Vaccination Notes: